THE COMPLETE

# CLINICAL

# MASSAGE

# THE COMPLETE GUIDE TO

# CLINICAL MASSAGE

**Christopher M. Norris**

BLOOMSBURY

LONDON • NEW DELHI • NEW YORK • SYDNEY

Published by Bloomsbury Publishing Plc
50 Bedford Square
London WC1B 3DP
www.bloomsbury.com

ISBN 978 1 4081 5457 1 (paperback)
ISBN 978 1 4081 8145 4 (ePDF)
ISBN 978 1 4081 8144 7 (EPUB)

**Acknowledgements**
Cover photograph © Shutterstock
Inside photographs © Laura Scott-Burns with the exception of Figure 3.8, p. 44 © Physique
Illustrations by David Gardner with the exception of Figures 7.2, 7.3 and 7.4 (pp. 112 and 113) © Jeff Edwards
Designed by James Watson
Typesetting and page layout by Susan McIntyre
Commissioned by Charlotte Croft
Edited by Nick Ascroft

Typeset in 10.75 on 14pt Adobe Caslon

Printed and bound in India by Replika Press Pvt. Ltd.

10 9 8 7 6 5 4 3 2 1

# CONTENTS

# INTRODUCTION

This book describes the practice of clinical massage, that is massage used to treat conditions such as injuries and pain known as 'clinical conditions' that are typically treated in a clinic. The methods described assume that the person applying the clinical massage (henceforth referred to as the therapist) has additional *clinical training* as a therapist or exercise professional.

We begin in chapters 1 and 2 by laying down important foundations of knowledge that deal with the process of tissues healing and injury recovery and the effect of massage on both these mechanisms and the body in general.

The book goes on to describe the effects of massage and in chapter 3 we look at traditional, or general, massage techniques, including effleurage, petrissage, tapotement, frictions and vibration/shaking, before going on in chapter 4 to describe specific clinical methods which target individual parts of the body, including fascial release (FR), deep tissue massage (DTM), trigger point (TrP) release, deep transverse friction (DTF), acupressure and muscle energy technique (MET).

We then look at how to plan a treatment session in chapter 5. It is important that the therapist is in possession of a diagnosis or clinical assessment indicating the tissues at fault (whether that be a ligament, muscle, etc.) and the mechanisms or pathology affecting the body (including swelling, pain, infection, etc.), and these areas are tackled in this chapter. Where the therapist is unsure of the diagnosis, treatment should not be carried out until the patient has contacted their GP (general practitioner) and determined whether there are reasons that clinical massage should not be used (known as a *contraindication*).

Chapters 6 to 9 are a compendium of massage techniques and exercises for you to use throughout your practice. Each chapter covers the most common techniques for every region of the body: the lower limbs, the trunk, the chest and abdomen and the upper limbs. The section includes an anatomy refresher for each region of the body, while over 90 massage techniques are demonstrated through photos and a detailed description of how to prepare and perform the massage. The section also includes tips and important points that will be valuable to your continued practice. Many of the techniques are performed with the client lying on a bench, which in clinical massage is more commonly called a treatment couch. However, for the purposes of this book the term 'bench' is used to describe this piece of equipment, as it will be a familiar term to all exercise professionals and, therefore, more inclusive.

The final chapter provides an overview of research into massage, which provides the scientific basis (known as the *evidence base*) for its use and purpose.

# MASSAGE IN PERSPECTIVE

1

Massage as a technique has its origins in a caring caress – after an injury, we rub the area that is in pain, while parents tell their children to 'rub it better' when they hurt themselves. Dogs lick themselves when they have an injury. The therapeutic value of touch has a place in all aspects of healthcare.

Historically, descriptions of massage and 'medical rubbing' have been found in most ancient civilisations. In Europe modern massage as a clinical technique can be traced back to the Swedish system of medical gymnastics (exercise applied for the treatment of medical conditions) founded by Ling in Stockholm, which spread across the world with institutes in both London and New York. Towards the end of the nineteenth century and beginning of the twentieth several books were published on massage in New York (Graham 1884), Germany (Hoffa 1897) and London (Goodall-Copestake 1926), which contributed to the wider popularity and understanding of massage's usage.

The formation in England of the Society of Trained Masseuses in 1895, the precursor of the Chartered Society of Physiotherapy, led to the standardisation of massage techniques and their quality and also the incorporation of massage into standard medical management. Further to this, the adoption of massage and soft tissue techniques by two hospital consultants, John Mennell (1920) and James Cyriax (1944) brought the benefits of this system to mainstream medical practice.

Massage has always straddled the border between art and science. The intuitive use of massage, using what 'feels right', must be balanced with the scientific proof that the techniques achieve what therapists claim they do. The instinctive nature of rubbing and intuitive use of therapeutic massage has led to its wide usage, but the evidence base for its benefits is sparse compared to other forms of treatment. This is partly because traditional massage had become an accepted form of treatment, applied to patients throughout history and often used almost without question. Although some early research was carried out – and is described in the books cited above – it is only with the spread in popularity of sports massage that modern research has started to accumulate in relation to this technique. Good quality evidence does exist, and we will refer to this throughout the book, but in many cases the experience of practitioners forms our guide. This should not belittle massage because its benefits are many.

Before we begin to outline the practice of clinical massage there are several theoretical principles which all practitioners should acquaint themselves with as a foundation for good practice.

# TYPES OF MASSAGE

A huge variety of massage types are available, with different 'shapes and flavours' of massage used in every culture across the world. These techniques can loosely be categorised into four major types: relaxation, clinical, re-education and energy work (*see* table 1.1). The categories are descriptive with much overlap existing between types.

## RELAXATION MASSAGE

*Relaxation* massage is used to help relieve stress and promote a general feeling of wellness. It is commonly used in spas and commercial gyms.

Sports massage falls into several categories and in this case relaxation techniques are used to prepare an athlete for competition. For example, in the case of a nervous or 'hyped' athlete muscle relaxation can calm them down and help them focus on their performance.

## CLINICAL MASSAGE

Clinical massage differs slightly from relaxation massage in that it promotes wellness, but rather it is used to specifically target something which is wrong with the body, for example a stiff arthritic knee joint, or to aid an individual in their recovery from injury, for example a torn ankle ligament. Again, sports massage can be used specifically to aid athletes in their recovering from a particular injury, for example a pulled hamstring muscle. In each case, massage can help by improving blood and lymph flow, warming and moving stiff tissues and reducing pain.

| Table 1.1 | Massage types | | | |
|---|---|---|---|---|
| **Type** | **Relaxation** | **Clinical** | **Re-education** | **Energy** |
| **Outcome** | • Relaxes client<br>• Promotes wellness | • Treats injury or clinical condition | • Use with movement | • Free blocked energy through *acupressure* or *meridians* (see boxes) |
| **Styles and techniques of massage** | • Swedish<br>• Aromatherapy<br>• Sports massage | • Fascial release<br>• Trigger point<br>• Transverse friction | • Muscle energy technique<br>• Passive stretching | • Acupressure<br>• Reflexology |

Norris, C. M. (2011) *Managing Sports Injuries* 4th edition (Elsevier)

## RE-EDUCATION MASSAGE

Re-education massage may be used with movement to correct movement faults (known as *dysfunction*). For example, massaging stiff tissue which is restricting movement. As the movement restriction is eased through massage application, correct movement is possible and exercise therapy can be applied to reinforce movement quality. Within clinical massage this type of re-education is common with techniques such as PNF stretching for example (*see* page 59), where muscles are tensed and then released to reduce their tone (firmness) and allow them to stretch more easily.

## ENERGY MASSAGE

Many massage techniques, from the East especially, are forms of *energy* massage. These include acupressure, which works to restore the flow of qi (life energy) through acupuncture channels or meridians (*see* 'Keypoint' box).

### Keypoint

In Traditional Chinese Medicine (TCM) qi energy is said to be transported throughout the body through a system of channels or *meridians*. Where the flow is blocked (which is known as qi stagnation) healing is poor and Chinese medicine believes that restoring the flow of qi will improve healing and reduce pain (see *also* chapter 6, page 103).

### Definition

*Acupressure* is a method of stimulating acupuncture points using finger pressure rather than needles (which is known as acupuncture).

## INJURY AND HEALING

Massage has most of its effect on the soft tissues of the body, rather than the bones. Soft tissues include the skin, muscles, fat, tendons, ligaments, nerves, internal organs and fascia (a thin fibrous membrane which surrounds other tissues such as muscles and ligaments, linking them together). When using clinical massage we may affect each of these tissues depending on the technique used.

### HOW INJURED TISSUE HEALS

Clinical massage is a technique often used following injury, and to be safe and effective as practitioners we need to understand how the body's tissues heal to enable us to work with the body's healing processes, rather than against them.

As healing progresses, your techniques may change, so knowledge of the healing timescale is also important to the therapist. The changes occurring within the healing tissues, and the parallel changes which you cause with massage treatment, must closely match if you are to achieve satisfactory treatment.

### Injury

The moment a client sustains an injury their tissues begin to heal. The process is continuous right up until the point where they have full function of the injured body part and can return to normal activities.

When soft tissue is damaged, some of the local blood capillaries running through it are disrupted, thus disturbing the release of fresh blood into the area. This has two important effects. Firstly, the tissue disruption instigates chemical messages to the brain that begin the healing process. Secondly, because the blood vessels are damaged, fresh blood can no longer flow into the local tissues. Starved of new blood, which should bring with it oxygen and tissue nutrients, the tissue begins to die. Think of this like watering your garden; if you cut the hose pipe, water cannot get to the flowers and they dry up and die. The same is true here, except it is a blood vessel which has been cut and your client's tissue rather than the flowers which may wither. If your client continues to exercise, the *metabolic rate* or 'tick over' of the tissues (*see* 'Definition' box) remains high and the demand for oxygen is increased. This increased demand speeds up tissue death, which is occurring due to the oxygen shortage. Rest is therefore vital to slow the metabolic rate and reduce the oxygen demand.

### Definition

*Metabolic rate* is the chemical 'tick over' of the body. It is the amount of oxygen and nutrients that your body requires just to keep going. Exercise increases metabolic rate while rest reduces it – much like putting your foot on a car accelerator pedal to use more petrol, and taking it off to use less.

Local cell death occurring in the injured tissues releases enzymes which begin the process of digesting and dissolving dead material. The body acts quickly as a natural 'road sweeper' to clean up the area in preparation for new tissue growth. This activity further stimulates the release of important chemicals including *histamine* and *prostaglandin*, which act as chemical messengers.

As blood escapes from the damaged blood vessels, red blood cells are in turn damaged by being outside their normal environment. The blood chemical *fibrin* then begins to form a meshwork around the injured area, which develops into a clot. The blood clot is an essential precursor to forming a bridge between the ends of the torn tissue, and any movement which disrupts the clot slows the normal healing process. Continuing to work hard or exercise in the immediate post-injury phase is therefore detrimental, as is the application of vigorous massage.

### Keypoint

Immediately after injury, tissues are disrupted and their blood flow reduced. Starved of new blood, tissue death will occur. Rest is vital to slow this process down.

### Inflammation

Inflammation begins 10 minutes after an injury occurs and may last several days depending on the first aid action which is taken. Inflammation gives four outward signs:

- 1. Heat
- 2. Redness
- 3. Swelling
- 4. Pain

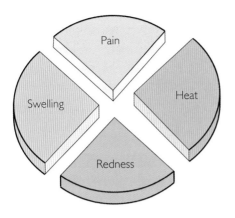

**Figure 1.1** Signs of inflammation

### Heat and redness

Both occur due to the increase in local blood flow, that is blood which flows close to the injured area. The increase develops as a result of blood vessels opening as a natural reaction to the injury. Just as your skin becomes red as you exercise and get hot, the local skin surrounding an injury reddens. However, this will only be noticeable where the damaged tissues are close to the surface (known as *superficial*). When your client sprains their ankle, the area feels hot and looks red, but if they damage their back, where the damaged tissues lie much deeper, the area may feel hot to you but to an outside observer redness is rarely noticeable unless the condition is very severe. Again the process of heat and reddening is brought about by a number of chemicals including *prostaglandin*. Anti-inflammatory drugs, such as *NSAIDs* (*see* 'Definition' box), are administered to calm the process of inflammation instigated by this chemical.

### Swelling

Broken blood vessels at the injury site cause blood flow to slow. The red blood cells become sticky and adhere to the vessel walls. The cells form part of the developing blood clot, which dams the area to stop further bleeding into the damaged tissues. *Swelling* (also called *oedema*) then begins as the slow blood movement is unable to keep pace with the fluids being formed by the body. As the damaged tissues release their chemicals, the body tries to dilute the area with watery fluid, which forms the basis of the swelling. The swelling moves into the lymphatic vessels and should be taken away as part of the normal lymph flow process (*see* 'Definition' box).

Unfortunately, the sheer volume of swelling which often develops after a soft tissue injury means that some will settle and pool around the injured area. Initially the swelling is a watery fluid, but it contains similar clotting chemicals to blood, and over time will become firmer and gel-like.

If left, over many weeks the gel-like swelling can harden still further. Clinical massage aims to remove excess swelling and stave off the problem of the tissue becoming stuck together (known as *consolidated oedema*). While massage helps the injury by removing swelling, if used too early or too vigorously it can disrupt the healing process and slow recovery.

### Pain

*Pain* is often the reason why many clients seek clinical massage. Pain following a soft tissue injury normally occurs because the chemicals produced at the time of injury irritate the nerve sensors within the tissues. As swelling occurs, the pressure of the developing fluids presses on these sensors and further pain is produced.

Pain is created by tiny electrical impulses travelling in nerves from the tissue sensors to the brain. This feeling (or *sensory*) mechanism consists of nerves which travel as a *pain pathway*, firstly to the spinal cord. Here, they form a junction (known as a *synapse*) with a small intermediate nerve (or *interneuron*) which itself connects to a longer fibre travelling to the brain where the pain is actually felt. Even within the brain there are several nerve connections (*see* figure 1.2).

At each junction between the nerves, the nerve impulse can be changed. This fact is important both for pain relief and for the development of longer term (or *chronic*) pain. If another nerve impulse arrives at the nerve junction in the spine, it can cancel out the painful signal. This is what happens when you knock your knee and 'rub it better' – the vigorous rubbing causes an intense sensory stimulus which cancels out the pain at the level of the spinal cord, an effect called *counterirritation* (*see* 'Definition' box).

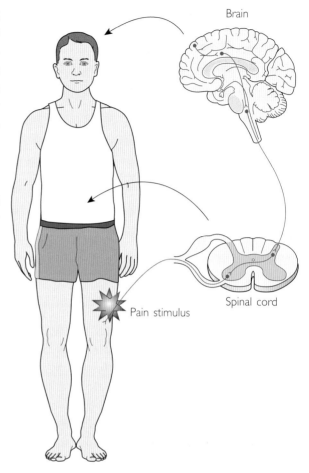

**Figure 1.2** The pain pathway

### Definition

A *counterirritant effect* is caused when a second intense stimulus cancels out a painful feeling. The effect occurs at the junction (or synapse) between two sensory nerves.

As the nerve impulse travels into the brain, you feel pain, a process that is known as sensory perception. However, the impulse also travels across junctions to other nerves going to different brain areas. Some go to emotional centres and so intense pain, especially if it occurs over a prolonged period, can cause emotional changes such as anxiety, fear and depression.

The nerve junctions can also work to your advantage. You can reduce or block pain by using many treatments, including clinical massage. Impulses produced by the brain as a result of treatment can flood the client's body with pain-relieving chemicals and have positive emotional effects.

## THE HEALING TIMESCALE

The process of tissue healing can take some time. Minor aches and pains may resolve in a matter of days, while more major problems can take many months and sometimes even years to heal completely. The key to the healing timescale is the amount of tissue damage your client has, and how the injury is treated. The process of healing described above proceeds through three interrelated phases: *acute*, *subacute* and *chronic*.

### Acute phase (48 hours)

During the acute phase your client's tissues have been damaged and are reacting to this through the stage of *inflammation*. There is local bleeding and swelling and the tissues will have only just started to heal. Your aim should be damage limitation – you must not take any action which stresses the damaged tissues and further injures the client. It is a sad fact that in some cases of sports injury, for example, there can be more tissue damage induced by trying to run an injury off than actually

occurred at the time of injury. In addition, we have seen that the swelling formed at the time of injury can spread throughout the local area. Limiting this spread is vital because the sticky swelling will clot, and if it travels this will affect further tissue.

The acute phase of healing typically lasts 48 hours and ceases when the tissues begin to form a healing bridge across the damaged area (*see* page 16). During this phase massage to the damaged tissues is not appropriate.

### Subacute phase (14–21 days)

When the healing tissues start to form and no fresh swelling or bleeding occurs, your client has entered the subacute phase of healing, which may last from anything between 14 and 21 days. This is the stage of *regeneration*, when tissue regrowth begins. Initially a soft blood clot forms and a stronger tissue mesh begins to grow around the area. The new healing tissue forms a scar in the same way that the skin heals after a cut. This tissue shrinks and pulls its torn ends together, effectively bridging the tissue gap. The tissue formed at this stage of healing is a meshwork fibres formed from fibrous tissue. Fibrous tissue contains two main types of fibres, one which is strong (fibrin) the other more elastic (elastin). The amount of each of these fibres is governed by the requirements of the tissue. For example both tendons (at the ends of muscles) and ligaments (at the side of joints) are made of fibrous tissue. However, ligaments are more stretchy than tendons and so have a greater proportion of elastin fibres than fibrin.

We have seen that after injury a blood clot forms (*see* figure 1.3a) and shrinks (figure 1.3b). The healing meshwork of fibrous tissue that begins to form has a haphazard, often known as *disorganised*, appearance, with fibres pointing in various directions (figure 1.3c). The finished tissue must have fibres which align in the strongest (known as *organised*) direction possible (figure 1.3d) and take on the function of the original tissue.

As your client's injury heals it is vital that their tissue remodels to closely resemble the original tissue format. If it is too loose or too tight, its function will be impaired. The make up of fibrous tissue changes depending on the stress placed upon it, and both massage and exercise have a role to play in ensuring the new tissue develops correctly. To change from the haphazard fibre orientation to a more organised mesh, the tissue must be stressed slightly. Too little stress and the fibres will not align correctly, but with too much stress

the fibres will break down again. In the subacute phase progressive massage and exercise are key. Massage when the client cannot perform a suitable movement, and prescribe exercise when they can.

## Chronic phase (21 days plus)

The final stage on the healing timescale is the chronic phase which is the stage of *remodelling* lasting from 21 days onwards. Although the term chronic is used here, this phase is an essential stage in which your client's scar tissue adapts to become more like the original tissue it has replaced. Both clinical massage and exercise therapy are useful now providing they place the correct amount of stress on the tissue. Too little will not stimulate remodelling, while too much can injure the tissues. The precise amount is judged by the client's reaction to treatment (*see* page 64). The remodelling phase can last for many years, and one of the mistakes which is often made during treatment is to stop the treatment too soon. Although your client's tissue may be relatively pain free when it has healed by 80 per cent, it has still not fully healed. Tissue at this stage can still break down when subjected to the stress of intense sport and it may give pain when subjected to prolonged postural loading, such as sitting for many hours at a computer.

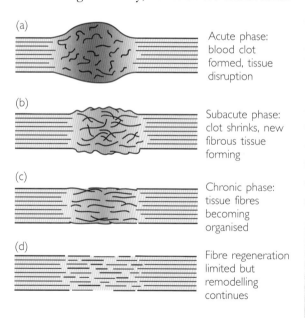

(a) Acute phase: blood clot formed, tissue disruption

(b) Subacute phase: clot shrinks, new fibrous tissue forming

(c) Chronic phase: tissue fibres becoming organised

(d) Fibre regeneration limited but remodelling continues

**Figure 1.3** A healing blood clot: (a) blood clot forms; (b) shrinks; (c) fibrous tissues form a disorganised meshwork; (d) the healed fibres must point in an organised direction

## Keypoint

During healing progressive massage and exercise are vital. Tissues must be stressed to encourage strong fibre development. The stress must match the strength of the newly formed tissue.

# THE EFFECTS OF MASSAGE

The effects of massage can be categorised into three areas: *physiological* (living processes), *biomechanical* (the physics of movement) and *psychological* (the mind and behaviour). All occur together, but for convenience we will look at them separately (*see* figure 1.4).

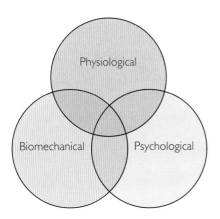

**Figure 1.4** The effects of massage

## PHYSIOLOGICAL EFFECTS OF MASSAGE

### Increasing blood flow

The effect of massage is to both increase blood flow to the skin and, through deeper techniques, to increase flow through the tissues beneath (the subcutaneous tissues). Greater blood flow means the speed of chemical reactions (such as metabolic rate) are increased. It is as though the tissues have been 'stirred up' so that everything happens faster.

Physiological effects are caused by the pressure of your hands on the skin compressing the blood and lymph vessels and so pressing fluid along them. As the pressure is released fluid can flow more easily, and the regular compression and release has a pumping effect on fluid flow. This effect can be aided by lifting (elevating) a limb above the level of the heart, as gravity will help to further increase fluid flow back towards the heart.

Blood flow is increased during clinical massage, both by the pumping effect of pressure described above and through skin stimulation. When the skin is struck sharply or pressed hard, it will go red and show slightly raised areas. This effect, known as the *triple response*, is an important way in which blood flow is increased. The triple response consists of an initial redness when the skin is stroked deeply. After a while this redness spreads causing a *flare* as blood flow increases around the stimulated area, due to blood vessels opening (known as *vasodilation*). Finally, a *weal* is produced where the skin puffs up as a result of the release of the blood chemical histamine. The combination of redness, flare and weal is the triple response.

> **Keypoint**
>
> The triple response is a skin (or *cutaneous*) reaction consisting of redness, flare and weal representing histamine release and consequent vasodilation.

### Hormonal changes

Hormonal changes also occur through massage, with research studies showing alterations in the hormones *cortisol*, *serotonin*, *dopamine* and *oxytocin*.

- *Cortisol* is a hormone produced by the adrenal glands sitting on top of the kidneys. It is released at times of stress and causes blood sugar levels to rise.

- *Serotonin* is a nerve chemical (neurotransmitter) which is produced in the gut wall and by nerves themselves. It has effects on mood, appetite and sleep especially.
- *Dopamine* is also a nerve chemical, but it is produced in the brain. It helps with many brain functions.
- *Oxytocin* is a sex hormone, and its concentration is changed by touch, stroking and hugging, especially in children.

Through these hormonal effects, massage can have positive effects on digestive processes, stress, anxiety levels and mood and sleep. In fact a client's wellness level can improve in general.

### Nerve impulses

The effect of massage on nerve impulses is also important. When we are anxious we often feel 'butterflies' in our stomach. This is an example of nerve impulses affecting the digestive system when we are under stress. Other ways that we feel stress include tightness around the neck and shoulder muscles. These are often called 'emotional muscles' because they are said to reflect our mood. A tense anxious person often has tight hunched shoulders. Muscles become tense because they are receiving a barrage of nerve impulses. Clinical massage can calm these impulses down and as a result relax tense muscles and ease muscle pain.

At the other extreme, weakened muscle has very few nerve impulses. Here, more vigorous massage can increase the number of impulses travelling into the muscle and help improve the tone of the muscle. It can also be used to help a client learn to tense (*contract*) muscle properly following a prolonged injury. In this

### Keypoint

Clinical massage may be used to either increase or reduce muscle tone depending on the technique chosen.

way, clinical massage can both increase or reduce muscle tone, depending on the precise technique selected.

## BIOMECHANICAL EFFECTS OF MASSAGE

The biochemical effects of clinical massage come mainly as a result of forces acting on the body tissues and the change in tissue temperature that massage can bring about. Five main forces are involved in clinical massage (*see* figure 1.5) and both the amount of force applied and the direction in which it is employed are important.

### Compression force

*Compression* (pressing) force may be applied rapidly with a tapping or cupping force or slowly with a *petrissage* (pressure) movement. Where a compressive force is applied using a small contact area, such as a fingertip, the effect on tissue is more marked than when the same force is applied using a broader area, such as the palm. High compressive forces rapidly applied over a small area may cause marked skin effects and even bruising if uncontrolled. Slower application over a broader area will cause fluid to flow away from the force. This can be repeated rhythmically to have a pumping effect to facilitate fluid flow through the tissues.

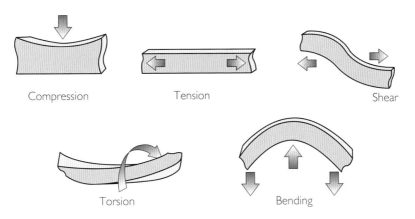

**Figure 1.5** The five main forces involved in clinical massage

## Tension force

*Tension* (pulling) forces occur when two ends of a structure are pulled apart. Sustained tension causes tissues to elongate and may be applied using drag and glide techniques on the skin and subcutaneous tissues. These involve pressing the fingers or palm into the tissues slightly to 'anchor' them and then pulling gently. Tension applied to muscle, known as *static stretch*, initially causes increased muscle tone and when sustained will cause muscle tension to gradually lower. Static stretch may be used as part of massage in the treatment of tight muscle or trigger points for example.

## Shear force

*Shear* (sliding) force occurs when the force is applied at an angle to the tissue, which creates a combination of both compression and stretch. This type of force may be used to encourage tissue layers to slide over each other. In addition shearing may be used to cause mild inflammation to restart the healing process where healing has stopped prematurely (a condition known as *stasis*) or the injury has not healed correctly. In this latter case shearing is used as a catalyst to restart healing which then takes place in parallel with gentle exercise therapy to encourage the tissues to continue to slide over each other and to avoid becoming fixed again.

## Torsion force

*Torsion* (twisting) force is used in wringing actions where your hands are gripping the client's tissues and turning in opposite directions. Torsion stretches the tissue in a rotary manner and may be used to enhance tissue pliability. Treatment using torsion may be applied where a tight band of tissue exists within surrounding normal tissue such as in scarring from a cut (superficial) or a healing muscle tear (deeper). The torsion force moves the stiffer scar tissue which would otherwise remain inactive as the surrounding tissues move instead.

## Bending force

*Bending* force combines compression on one side of a tissue and elongation on the other to create a concave and convex shape respectively. Again, tissue pliability is improved through use of this technique.

### How does the application of force help healing?

The application of a force causes changes within tissue because the tissues are *thixotropic*. Thixotropy is a property of certain materials which are normally quite stiff (they have high *viscosity*) to become more fluid and flow (to have low viscosity) when agitated or subjected to physical stress.

A typical example of thixotrophy is children's modelling clay. When a child begins to play with clay it is stiff and hard, but as they work it with their hands it becomes softer and more malleable, making it easier to shape.

## Keypoint

Many human tissues are thixotrophic. In their normal state they are quite stiff, but when massaged they become more fluid and mobile.

Stimulation of the healing tissue through the mechanical loading of massage (or exercise) results in *mechanotransduction* (Khan & Scott 2009), a mechanism by which a mechanical stimulus is converted into electrical and/or chemical signals. The process has three interrelated components: *mechanocoupling*, *cell-to-cell communication* and *effector cell response*.

Mechanocoupling is the method through which forces created through massage such as shear, compression and tension, deform tissue cells and are transformed into chemical signals. The effect of cell deformation is not restricted to the local area of massage however. Through the process known as cell-to-cell communication, signals are conducted from the massaged area throughout the wider tissue region. At the points

## Definition

A *gap junction* is a very fine communication channel between cells. Also called nanotubes, gap junctions allow chemicals to pass from one cell to another through the outer cell membrane. A gap junction effectively connects the jelly interior (cytoplasm) of one cell with the other.

where cells touch each other *gap junctions* are formed (*see* 'Definition' box).

Various chemicals including calcium and inositol triphosphate pass through these so that cells can communicate with each other directly. In reality it is only certain forms of these chemical which pass through. These forms (called ions) are charged electrically and can be affected by electrical forms of therapy used in hospitals to treat injured tissues.

Finally, this chemical message causes a tissue change called an *effector cell response*. *Integrins* (receptors on the outside of the cell) form a bridge between the *extracellular region* (outside of the cell) and the *intercellular region* (inside of the cell). The *cytoskeleton* of the cell (the cell's 'skeleton', formed from protein and present in all cells) sends a direct physical stimulus to the cell nucleus, and biochemical signals (called *gene expression*) are caused by the integrins. As a result the cell nucleus gives a signal to begin protein synthesis and the new protein is secreted into the extracellular matrix, causing it to remodel. The massage we give causes direct chemical changes such as this, which promotes the repair and remodelling of the injured tissues.

Clinical massage draws blood into the tissues being treated and the tissue temperature rises.

> ## Keypoint
>
> Through the process of mechanotransduction, massage can cause direct chemical changes that promote tissue repair.

This rise in temperature will speed up the natural chemical reactions which occur within the tissues and as a result contribute to speeding the healing process itself.

## PSYCHOLOGICAL EFFECTS OF MASSAGE

### Arousal level

Psychological effects occur as a result of arousal and the effects of anxiety and stress. Arousal level is particularly important when applying clinical massage in sport. It is intimately linked to performance and this can be shown graphically on the arousal-performance curve (inverted-U curve, *see* figure 1.6). When a client is under-aroused they will be lethargic and perform poorly. As their arousal level increases they will be more motivated and alert, so their performance is likely to improve. However, an over-aroused client will be nervous and too 'psyched up'. As a consequence their performance will suffer. Ideally the client should be at the centre of the arousal-performance curve so that their performance is optimal.

Assessing the arousal level of a client prior to using clinical massage in sport is therefore vital. Clinical massage can be used to stimulate the under-aroused individual, but calm those who are over-aroused. Stimulating an already highly aroused nervous individual will push them too

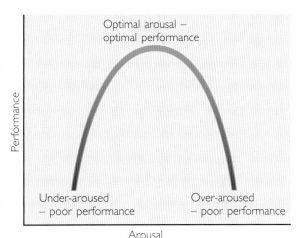

**Figure 1.6** The arousal-performance curve

far to the right of the arousal-performance curve, while relaxing an under-aroused client will have the opposite effect.

### Mood level

Clinical massage can also have an important psychological effect on a client's *mood*. From a psychological perspective, mood is defined as a long-lasting emotional effect. Someone may flare up and be angry, for example when demonstrating an emotion, but over time their type of mood or 'mood state' may change to become more permanent. Common mood states include anxiety, depression, fatigue, anger, vigour and confusion. Clinically, mood state is often measured using a test called the profile of mood states (POMS), but from the perspective of clinical massage it is sufficient to judge if a client has a positive or negative mood by talking to your client and observing their general response to your questions.

Massage has been shown to have positive effects on mood state, improving a person's mood, particularly where mood is associated with long term illness.

# CONTRAINDICATIONS AND CAUTIONS TO CLINICAL MASSAGE

*Contraindications* are conditions that a client may have which make clinical massage unsuitable. *Cautions* indicate that massage should only be used with care and continual reassessment of the client (*see* table 1.2). Both contraindications and cautions fall into one of two categories, *systemic* and *topical*. Systemic factors affect the whole body or multiple parts of the body (organs, joints, tissues) while topical factors are localised to a single area.

## SYSTEMIC INFECTION

The infection may be something as simple as flu, or may be an active condition such as MRSA within a hospital. The danger is that clinical massage, due to its effect on speeding the metabolic rate, may increase the severity of the disease, or tax the body unnecessarily when the body needs to focus on combating the disease.

## ACUTE STAGE OF INJURY

The effect on the metabolic rate is also the reason why massage is contraindicated at the acute stage of a soft tissue injury. As the injury moves into the subacute phase, massage is helpful to aid in swelling removal. The key here is that although swelling is present, it is not fresh swelling formed by active inflammation, but old swelling which has remained within the tissues.

## CROSS-INFECTION

The danger of cross-infection between clients, or between the therapist and client, means that massage over an open wound or local skin infection, however small, is contraindicated. Wounds on either the client or therapist should be covered with a sterile waterproof dressing, even if they are not within an area to be massaged, as cross-infection may still occur due to air movement.

## BLOOD THINNING MEDICATION

Certain drugs such as Warfarin act as anticoagulants to stop blood clotting by thinning the blood. As certain intense massage techniques can sometimes cause minor bruising or vein breakage, it is contraindicated when clients are on this medication. If minor bleeding were to occur into the tissues, effective blood clotting and tissue repair may be slowed.

## MYOSITIS OSSIFICANS

This is a condition where deep bruising from a very bad knock in sports such as rugby can release bone-forming cells (*osteoblasts*) into the area. As a result, the bruised area can harden and calcify with bone crystals being laid down. Where this is likely, massage is contraindicated as it may spread the bone forming cells, causing more extensive tissue disruption. Where deep bruising is present, especially over the front of the thigh (quadriceps muscles) or front of the arm (biceps muscle), medical guidance should be sought before massage is given.

## ALTERED SKIN SENSATION

Massage affects sensors within the skin which are responsible for feeling (*sensory nerve endings*). As such, if the skin sensation is reduced the client will not be able to feel the pressure of the massage and give feedback about excessive pressure and pain. Sensory loss of this type can occur through nerve entrapment or damage

| Table 1.2 | Contraindications and cautions to clinical massage |
| --- | --- |
| **Contraindication/caution** | **Reason as to why clinical massage may not be suitable** |
| Systemic infection | Infection is affecting the whole body |
| Acute stage of injury | Inflammation is still forming |
| Open wound | Wound is within the massage site |
| Circulatory condition | The condition of the skin may be poor and easily damaged by massage techniques |
| Infectious skin condition | Danger of cross-infection |
| Blood thinning medication | Seek medical guidance |
| Myositis ossificans | Recent direct bruising to thigh or anterior arm |
| Altered skin sensation | Seek medical guidance |
| Deep vein thrombosis (DVT) | If recovered within three months, still seek medical guidance |
| Directly over tumour | Massage used extensively within oncology (the branch of medicine that deals with cancer), but seek medical guidance |

following low back pain or neck whiplash, for example. Until the skin sensation has returned massage should not be used except by a qualified physiotherapist who can assess the extent of nerve damage.

## DEEP VEIN THROMBOSIS (DVT)

Deep vein thrombosis (DVT) is the formation of a blood clot within a deep vein. It occurs particularly within the deep vein of the leg and calf (femoral vein and or popliteal vein). The leg can appear red, swollen and painful with the superficial veins (close to the body surface) becoming overloaded and engorged. Where this occurs the patient should seek medical guidance. The danger of a DVT is that part of the clot may break loose and travel to the lungs, where it can form a pulmonary embolism. This can lead to severe chest pain, difficulty in breathing and eventually lung collapse. The condition can be fatal. Clearly there is a risk that massage may dislodge part of the DVT causing a pulmonary embolism. It should therefore not be used under any circumstances.

## DIRECTLY OVER A TUMOUR

A tumour is a solid lesion (lump) formed by excessive cell growth and is also termed a *neoplasm*, meaning 'new growth'. It can occur where cancer is present in the tumour (*malignant*), but importantly many tumours are non-cancerous (known as *benign*).

Because massage speeds the metabolic rate, there is a risk in theory that it may increase the spread of cells. Although massage directly over a tumour is contraindicated, clinical massage is used extensively and with marked effect within hospital oncology (cancer) units where it aids in treatment recovery and enhances well-being. However, it should be performed under medical guidance.

## Keypoint

Tumours may be benign or malignant. Benign tumours do not (a) grow in a rapid and uncontrolled manner, (b) move into (invade) surrounding tissues and (c) spread to other non-related areas of the body (*metastasise*).

## Summary of key terms

- **Anticoagulants** Chemical which stops blood clotting
- **Contraindications** Conditions a client may have which make clinical massage unsuitable
- **Cortisol** Hormone produced by the adrenal glands, which are located on top of the kidneys
- **Dopamine** Nerve chemical produced in the brain

- **Fibrin** Blood chemical involved in clotting
- **Histamine** Chemical messenger
- **Oedema** Medical term for swelling
- **Oxytocin** Sex hormone
- **Pathology** Something which is wrong with the body
- **Prostaglandin** Chemical messenger
- **Serotonin** Nerve chemical
- **Synapse** Nerve junction

# CLINICAL MASSAGE PREPARATION

Before you apply clinical massage, there is some preparation to be done. We need to look at how you are going to use your hands and how to maintain the correct posture when massaging. We are also concerned with the positioning of your client, and the contact medium you use between your hands and your client's skin. These subjects lay the foundation for good clinical practice.

## YOUR BODY

Massage is traditionally carried out with the therapist's hands. However, there are other areas of the body which can be used and methods of hand usage which can reduce the strain on the hands. This is important because many massage therapists suffer injuries to their hands due to performing treatments day-to-day. A study by the Chartered Society of Physiotherapy in the UK looked at 3600 physiotherapists who use there hands daily in patient treatments. It found that a high percentage had suffered from repetitive strain injuries (RSI). Revealingly the percentage was higher in recently qualified and less experienced staff, suggesting that both training and experience were important factors in the outcome. Similar studies in the United States and Australia have found comparable results, with up to 91 per cent of recently qualified therapists complaining of musculoskeletal pain due to their job (Cromie et al. 2000). The key to preventing therapist injuries is to learn methods of applying clinical massage with the least stress imposed on your own body.

As a therapist performing clinical massage, you are applying a force to your client through a point of contact. The point of contact may be your hand, fingers, elbow, forearm or another area. Importantly, the point of contact does not create the force, but merely transmits it. The force itself is created by your body weight.

This process of separating the creation and transmission of a force is not unique to clinical massage. Let's take an example from sport. Someone practising martial arts may be able to break a brick with their bare hand. Yet, we know that a brick dropped onto the bare hand might

### Keypoint

Use your hands and fingers to transmit, rather than create, the massage force.

actually break the bones in the hand. So how does the martial artist break the brick rather than their hand? The answer is that they use their body to create the force needed to break the brick, especially through movement of the hips and pelvis, and their hand to apply the force for a very small period of time. By tightening all of the hand muscles and making the hand into a single unit, this brief period of intense force creates a spike in pressure on the brick causing it to crack. The key is to combine a brief force application through a very stable hand which has been reinforced by muscle action. This intelligent use of the body is something we should aim for in the application of clinical massage.

## YOUR FINGERS

Everyone is different – tall, short, fat, thin. The same is true for your hands. Some therapists have long slender fingers, while others have short and stout ones. If your fingers are shorter and stronger you will be able to apply great power but may lack dexterity. Those with slender, more delicate fingers may have good dexterity but are also more open to hand injuries. When you apply powerful techniques in clinical massage it is essential that your fingers remain stable. Fingers which bend too much (known as *hyperflexible*) place greater stress on the finger tissues (*see* figure 2.1). It is important to avoid these excessive movements on the fingers by supporting your finger joints, or using alternative contact methods.

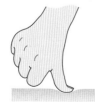

**Figure 2.1**
Hyperextending fingers

## Single finger

One finger used on its own is quite delicate and likely to be injured unless the amount of force used is very small. Bend (flex) your finger slightly and tighten your finger muscles to protect the joints. As you press on the finger it will straighten slightly, but if you start with it straight, it may hyperextend when loaded (*see* figure 2.2). The single finger is used on small body structures such as the lumbrical muscles between your client's toes or fingers. Where small regions are to be treated but more pressure is to applied, support one finger with another.

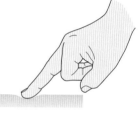

**Figure 2.2**
Single finger

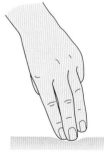

**Figure 2.3**
Normally the index finger and third finger are used as a single unit

## Supported finger

Normally the index finger and third finger are used as a single unit (*see* figure 2.3), each bent slightly so that the two fingertips are level. The pad of the index finger is now used as the massage tool. Where body weight is used to press through the supported finger, using it as a 'spear', be careful to align the finger bones (phalanges) hand bones (metacarpals)

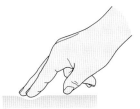

**Figure 2.4** Use two or three fingers to form a ridge to apply pressure

and forearm bones (radius especially). Where a straight line is formed through these three units any body weight used will be transmitted directly through the bones to the point of application (finger pad). If the bones are not aligned, some of the force will be lost, causing the joints to bend and stressing the supporting soft tissues. One or two fingers (*see* figure 2.4) may be combined to form a 'ridge' to apply pressure along a line.

## KNUCKLE

The knuckle may be used where greater force is applied, for example when releasing a trigger point (*see* chapter 4). The knuckle itself (metacarpal phalangeal or 'MCP' joint) or first finger joint (proximal interphalangeal or 'PIP' joint) may be used with the contact area flat or more prominent (*see* figure 2.5). Where a larger area is required, the whole fist can be used. Be careful not to allow your knuckle to dig into your client's tissues. Ease off pressure when you are directly over a bone area and increase pressure when you move onto thicker soft tissues.

## FIST

Using the fist enables more body weight to be used without endangering the finger joints.

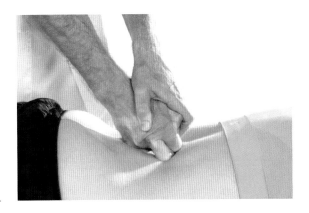

**Figure 2.5** The knuckle itself or first finger joint may be used with the contact area flat or more prominent

However, this is a powerful technique and should be used with caution over fleshy areas. Thin or delicate tissue and prominent bone areas should again be avoided. Where force is used by leaning onto the knuckle, fist or elbow, there is always the risk of slipping and causing a skin burn on your client. For this reason the web space of your other hand should be used to frame the area (*see* figure 2.6). The side of the fist may be used in traditional massage striking (percussion) techniques, which is known as *beating*.

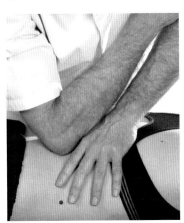

**Figure 2.6** Use the web space of your hand to frame the area to avoid your knuckles or elbow slipping, which could cause skin burn on your client

## PISIFORM

The pisiform is a small pea shaped bone on the little finger side of the wrist. It is actually a *sesamoid* bone (*see* 'Definition' box) lying within the tendon of the flexor carpi ulnaris (FCU) muscle in the forearm. The pisiform creates a joint with the ulna (inner forearm bone) and triquetral, a wrist bone lying below the fifth finger.

> ### Definition
>
> A *sesamoid* is a small bone embedded within a tendon which passes close to a joint. By holding the tendon away from the joint slightly, the sesamoid protects the tendon and acts as a pivot point increasing the leverage effect (mechanical advantage) of the tendon. The most widely known sesamoid is the kneecap (patella), lying within the quadriceps tendon.

By flexing the wrist and tilting it sideways towards the thumb (radial deviation) the pisiform becomes prominent and may be used as a powerful massage tool (*see* figure 2.7). Its size approximates to that of a fingertip, but the skin over the area of your pisiform is less sensitive than that over your fingertips, making the pisiform better for power techniques rather than fine movements.

## HYPOTHENAR EMINENCE

The hypothenar eminence is the pad on the little finger side of the hand, the thenar eminence being the pad on the thumb side of the arm. Both may be used as broad contact areas to apply either static pressure or to slide across tissues to create

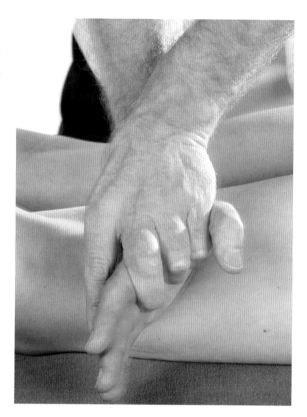

**Figure 2.7** By flexing the wrist and tilting it sideways towards the thumb the pisiform becomes prominent and can be a powerful massage tool

friction or tissue shearing force (*see* figure 2.8a). They are often used bilaterally in an X-grip action (*see* figure 2.8b) .

## HEEL OF HAND

The heel of the hand consists of the thenar eminence and the end of both the radius (forearm bone) and scaphoid bone. This whole region can be used to create very large amounts of force where the whole body weight is leant forwards onto the hand. Evidence of its power is the fact that the heel of the hand is often used to manipulate in therapy and as a deadly strike

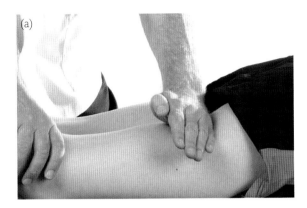

(a)

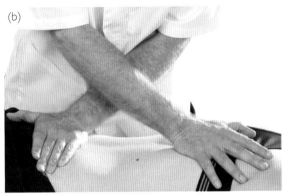

(b)

**Figure 2.8** Using the hypothenar eminence (the pad on the little finger side of the hand): (a) to create friction or tissue shearing force; (b) bilaterally in an X-grip action

in martial arts (in a palm heel strike) (*see* figure 2.9). One word of caution however; if you have very slender wrists, the amount of power you can create by leaning forwards can stress your wrist excessively. If this occurs, consider using a wrist support (splint) or ensure that you support your wrist with your other hand whenever you use power techniques in clinical massage.

## FOREARM

The forearm offers a broad contact area particularly suited to effleurage (*see* page 38) and fascial stretching (*see* page 48) over large areas of skin on the back and the back of the thigh (hamstrings), for example. The upper part of the forearm gives a softer general contact area, the lower part a sharper ridge which can be used to direct force in a more focused way. In addition, the forearm can be rolled (*pronation* and *supination*) over tissue to create a combination of pressure and motion (*see* figure 2.10). However, remember to wash this area when you have finished applying clinical massage. Many therapists wash their hands following treatment, forgetting that other areas of their skin may have been in contact with their client.

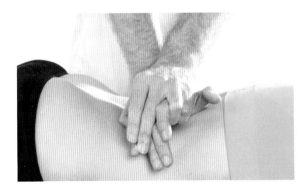

**Figure 2.9** A palm heel compression can be used to create a large amount of force

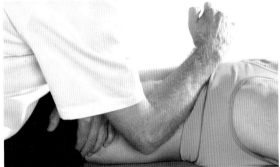

**Figure 2.10** The forearm can be rolled over tissue to create a combination of pressure and motion

29

## ELBOW

The elbow gives a relatively small but powerful focused area, which is especially suited to trigger point release. As with the fist above, as you lean your body weight onto the region there is a tendency to slip across the skin surface, so the web space of your other hand should be used to frame the area (*see* figure 2.11). From the therapist point of view there is one word of caution here; the ulnar nerve runs within a small groove at the inner part of the elbow, so pressure should be placed at the point of the elbow (olecranon) rather than the inner edge (medical epicondyle).

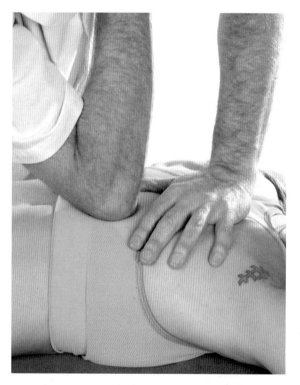

**Figure 2.11** When using your elbow, remember to use the web space of your hand to frame the area

### Keypoint

When applying pressure through the elbow, avoid the inner aspect to protect the delicate ulnar nerve.

## COMMERCIAL MASSAGE TOOLS

A number of massage tools are available to the therapist. These may be used as an extension to your hands and allow you to apply greater pressure to your client without endangering your finger joints and tissues (*see* figure 2.12).

### THE INDEX KNOBBLER

The index knobbler is a T-shaped plastic or wooden tool which is held in the hand. The ball of the tool may be used to provide deep focused pressure, which is useful when targeting trigger points. The side of the tool provides a ridge-like surface which can be used to cover wider areas. By forming the hand into a fist when applying pressure rather than using the open fingers or thumbs, this type of device enables your wrist to be locked and fingers protected.

The Superthumb is a sprung version of the knobbler which is used by physiotherapists to apply highly localised pressure when performing joint mobilisation or trigger point release. The tip of the tool is rubber, which does not slip, and the end is interchangeable in three different sizes. The Superthumb tool has been subjected to scientific evaluation to compare it to using the hands to apply joint mobilisation to the lumbar spine. The ability of the physiotherapist to feel changes in

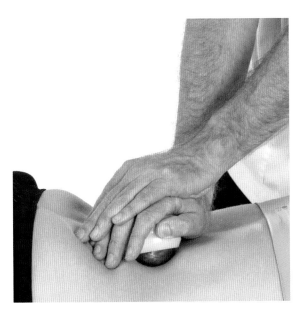

**Figure 2.12** There are a number of massage tools that can be used as an extension to your hands

the lumbar joints (known as *tactile feedback*) was comparable to using a pisiform contact with their hands. However, the Superthumb tool was perceived as less comfortable by patients than the physiotherapists hands (Maher et al. 2002).

## THE JACKNOBBER

The Jacknobber has several similar tips to the index knobbler that vary in size. Shaped like a toy jack it is easy to grip, and the different tip sizes ensure that the correct contact area is used for a specific tissue.

## TENNIS/GOLF BALL/EGG

For focused pressure a firm tennis ball or golf ball may be used, and the egg is a commercial equivalent to this. Shaped like a hen's egg, it is either made from plastic or stone and can be held in the cupped hand. The stone version may be

heated with hot water or cooled by soaking in iced water to provide additional local stimulation.

## THERAPIST'S THUMB

The Therapist's Thumb is an ergonomically shaped plastic deep tissue massage tool. You grip the ridged edge of the tool in your hand and place your thumb in the cup formed by the shallow end of the tool. Deep pressure can be applied without stress on your thumb joint, which is particularly important if this joint has a tendency to hyperextend.

## VIBRATORY MASSAGE MACHINES

Vibratory massage machines are useful where intense shaking, vibration or percussion is given. These range from hand-held lightweight devices to commercial free-standing units which have their motor separate to their application head. In this way power is provided without the need to lift and hold a heavy machine. In sport, vibratory massage is often claimed to offset fatigue. However, there is little scientific evidence for this being successful. An early study over 20 years ago confirmed this (Cafarelli et al. 1990). It looked at quadriceps contraction to fatigue (70 per cent maximum voluntary contraction or MVC, that is the peak force produced by a muscle as it contracts while pulling against an immovable object) in male athletes. The study authors found that there was no difference in how quickly the quadriceps muscles fatigued between those receiving vibration therapy (experimental group) and those who did not (control group). A more recent study compared the effect of Swedish massage and vibratory massage on the recovery of post-surgical patients and found no difference between the two types (Taylor et al. 2003).

## POSTURE AND BODY MECHANICS WHEN APPLYING TECHNIQUES

Your hands are not the only body part which can be stressed when applying massage. Tension around the shoulders from a rounded shoulder (known as *protracted*) is common among therapists, as is low back pain from prolonged back bending (*lumbar flexion*).

To avoid excessive stress on your own body, begin by making sure the bench you are working on is at the right height for you. For firm pressure you will want to press through straight arms and so the bench should be at about your mid-thigh level. For normal clinical massage have the bench at hip height, and lower your own height by bending your knees slightly rather than leaning over. Aim to keep your breastbone (sternum) more or less vertical rather than pointing it down towards the bench.

### Keypoint

When using firm pressure, press through straight arms and have your treatment bench at mid-thigh level. For normal clinical massage have the bench at about hip height.

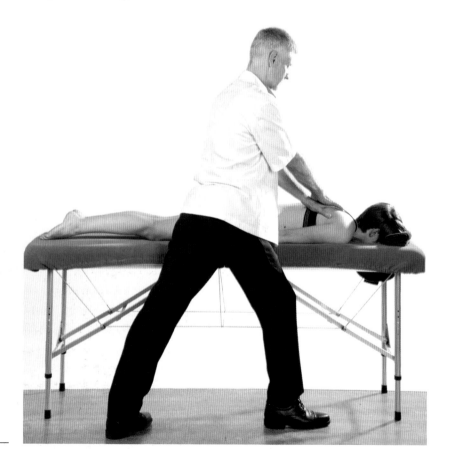

**Figure 2.13a** Massage stance positions: walk standing

When producing power for clinical massage techniques, the power should come from your legs and hips. Take a stance with one foot forwards, known as *walk standing* (*see* figure 2.13a), when facing the top or bottom of the bench to give longitudinal movements. Use a wide stance, known as *stride standing* (*see* figure 2.13b), when facing the sides for lateral movements or short-range longitudinal actions. For larger longitudinal movements transfer your weight from your back foot to your front, pressing your hips forwards. For lateral movements shift your hips back and forwards, taking your weight over your heels and then leaning into the bench, with your weight over your toes. As a self-check your pelvis should face your direction of movement. In this way you avoid twisting your spine.

Deliver the power for the massage stroke through your arms and hands, keeping your elbows and wrists locked. Allowing these joints

## Keypoint

When you performing clinical massage while standing, place your pelvis in the direction of movement to avoid excessive twisting of your spine.

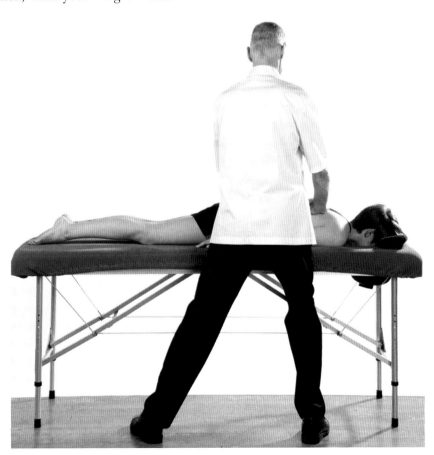

**Figure 2.13b** Massage stance positions: stride standing

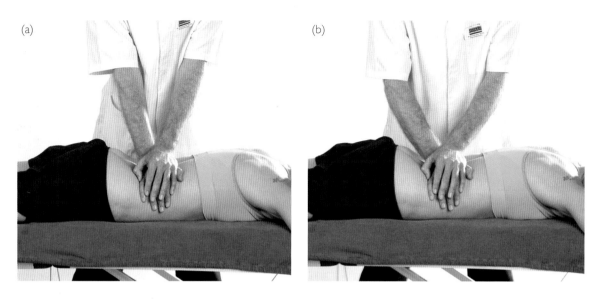

(a)

(b)

**Figure 2.14** Allowing your elbows and wrists to bend will result in some power being lost so you will have to work harder

to bend will result in some of the power being lost so you will have to work harder (*see* figure 2.14) .

Make sure that you do not over-reach. You should feel relatively relaxed when applying massage. If you are straining or holding your breath, you are doing something wrong. Move closer to the treatment bench and relax your shoulders. Use rhythmical body sway as you apply the techniques, transferring body weight and timing your strokes so you have a chance to recover, using an on-off action when applying force. Continual pressure or gripping actions will exhaust your own muscles, leading to acids accumulating in them (lactate build-up), which may cause aching and burning. Allowing the muscles to relax and recover between massage strokes allows fresh blood to enter the area (known as *blood perfusion*), which brings oxygen to the working muscles and flushes waste products away.

## MASSAGE MEDIUM

Most massage techniques have to strike a balance between holding the tissues to manipulate them, which is known as 'grip', and sliding across the tissues to stimulate them, which is known as 'slip'. Grip (friction) is needed to lift the tissues in petrissage techniques (*see* page 40) and to move the fingers and skin as a single unit in *deep transverse friction* (DTF) techniques (*see* chapter 4). In both of these cases if your hands slip over your client's skin surface while you are applying a forceful technique, it may result in friction damage to their skin. To avoid this wipe your client's skin with a paper towel or alcohol wipe if they have very oily or moist skin. Also consider using talc or resin to enhance your grip.

Where some glide is required, but your clinical massage technique is still quite forceful and localised (for example, when undertaking deep tissue work) use a thicker massage wax.

Where you need to slide over a wider area, use an oil-based cream or body oil. Some of this product will be absorbed into the client's skin, so ensure you reapply the product regularly.

Many sports massage oils are based on mineral oil. This consists of large particles which lie on the surface of the skin rather than being fully absorbed into the skin. Some clinical massage oils consist of a mixture of base oil which may be plant-based with essential plant oils added. Base oils include such products as grapeseed and nut oils such as almond. Essential oils also have medicinal properties and include products such as tea tree and chamomile (which is an antiseptic). Mixing essential oils for a client is a specialist technique in aromatherapy massage and requires specific training. The Chartered Society of Physiotherapy has a professional network for specialist physiotherapist working in this area. They can be contacted via their website www.csp.org.uk/professional-networks/cpmastt. The Federation of Holistic Therapies (FHT) has information on courses and publications again accessed via their website at www.fht.org.uk.

## CLIENT POSITIONING

Your client must be positioned so they feel supported and secure. If they feel they may fall or turn, they will tense themselves and make the massage harder to conduct.

### CLIENT ON THEIR FRONT

When the client is on their front, either use a bench with a breathing slot or roll/fold a towel

### Keypoint

Your massage medium has to strike a balance between high friction (grip) and low friction (slip).

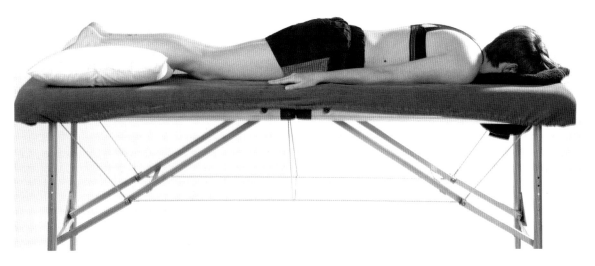

**Figure 2.15** This shows the client correctly positioned on their front

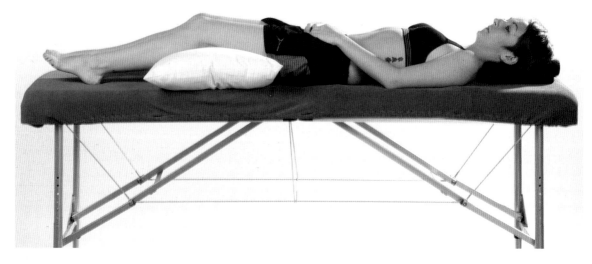

**Figure 2.16** This shows the client correctly positioned on their back

and place it beneath their forehead. In each case this will avoid squashing their nose and impeding breathing. If you do place something under their forehead, however, make sure it is not so big as to thrust their head backwards (cervical extension). When lying on their front female clients are often more comfortable with a soft cushion or pillow beneath their breasts, and most clients appreciate a roll under their shins to release tension at the back of the knee (the *popliteal region*).

## CLIENT ON BACK

When on their back, clients should have a roll beneath their knees and a support of some sort under their head. Those with round shoulders and upper spine (increased thoracic kyphosis) will need a thicker support to avoid their head falling back into extension. Some older clients find lying flat for a prolonged period difficult because they can get breathless (a medical condition called

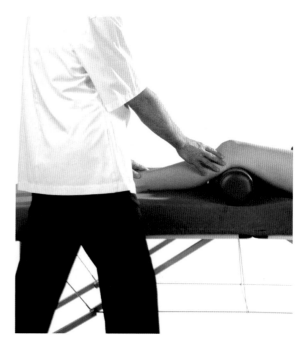

**Figure 2.17** This shows the client correctly positioned for focus on one limb

*orthopnea*). For these clients use a bench with a chest section which can be raised to 20–30 degrees, or prop them up on pillows or cushions to the same angle.

## FOCUSING ON ONE LIMB

Where one limb is the focus of massage, it must be relaxed and supported. Placing a foam rubber block (yoga pad), roll or folded towel beneath the client's shin, for example, will enable the heel to raise from the bench surface and the ankle joint to be moved freely. Supporting the client's arm over the therapists thigh (protected by a towel) can provide sufficient stability for massage within the sporting environment where little equipment is at hand.

## FORWARD LEAN SITTING

If your client is unable to lie down, they may be treated sitting and leaning forward (forward lean sitting) on a supporting surface such as the treatment bench or even an office desk. They should sit on a chair or low stool facing the bench with their feet comfortably apart. Place two pillows on the bench in front of them and allow them to rest their forearms on the pillows. Raise the bench (or stack the pillows higher if it is a fixed height bench or desk) so that your client's back is not rounded (flexed), but not so high that their shoulders shrug. Commercially available massage chairs and bench top supports (*see* figure 2.18) may also be used. These have

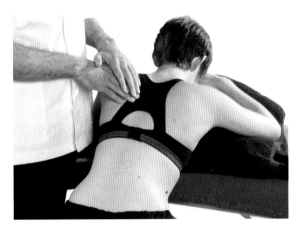

**Figure 2.18** This shows the client correctly positioned in forward lean sitting

the advantage that they are adjustable, and the massage chairs allow your client to sit with their knees lower than their hips, a more comfortable position for the lower (lumbar) spine.

### Summary of key terms

- **Hyperflexible** Joint which bends more than the average
- **Longitudinal movement** Movement in line with the long side edge of a treatment bench
- **Lateral movement** Movement across a bench in line with the short edge
- **Repetitive strain injuries (RSI)** Injuries caused by repeated movement

# TRADITIONAL MASSAGE TECHNIQUES

**3**

At its most basic level, massage can be viewed as simply a modification of the stroking which parents instinctively use on their children, or the rubbing which we all apply to ourselves when we knock into something. We can categorise therapeutic rubbing into five main movements, some traditionally described using French names and, in the UK and Dutch speaking countries, collectively known as Swedish massage (elsewhere they are known as classical or traditional massage). They were first popularised and taught in a systematic form by Per Henrik Ling in Sweden and Johan Georg Mezger in Holland and are known as:

- 1. Effleurage
- 2. Petrissage
- 3. Tapotement
- 4. Frictions
- 5. Vibration/shaking

## 1. EFFLEURAGE

Effleurage is a stroking action performed with the flat of your hands. True effleurage is a movement away from the therapist, leading with the fingers, while stroking is a movement towards the therapist leading with the heel of the hand. The techniques are often used to start and finish a massage and to spread massage oil or cream, but would not be used on broken skin which may become irritated or infected.

## TECHNIQUE

The flat of either one or both of your hands is normally used, but any flat surface can apply effleurage (*see* figure 3.1). The side and front of your forearm is a useful massage tool for effleurage which takes stress off the wrist and hand (*see* figure 3.2).

When applying effleurage, rather than pressing with your hand, lean forwards slightly keeping your elbows locked and press into the skin. To avoid digging into the skin, either keep your fingers straight and massage inline with the fingers, or contour the limb with your hand and lead with the side of your hand or webspace. Press evenly and move slowly. To help with this imagine how it would feel to press water out of a sponge. You can press quickly and the water will spurt out. Now imagine that you are pressing oil out of the sponge instead – you will need to press slowly to allow the oil to flow steadily. This is the type of feeling you should get when applying effleurage; a slow flowing movement to encourage tissue fluid to move beneath your hands.

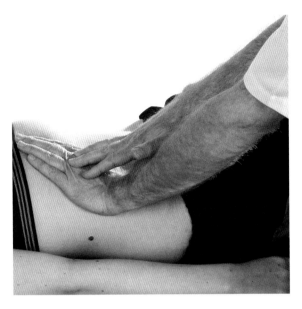

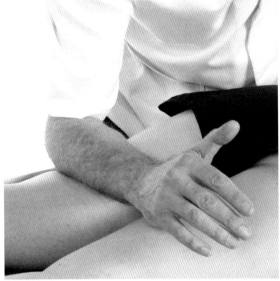

**Figure 3.1** Any flat surface can apply effleurage

**Figure 3.2** You can use the forearm to apply effleurage

As you get to the end of your effleurage stroke, release the pressure and relax your hand as you return it to the start position. In this way your hand and arm gets a chance to recover between strokes.

For deeper effleurage the direction of the stroke is always towards the centre of the chest, so foot to thigh or hand to shoulder. This is the direction in which the lymph fluid flows through its vessels towards the heart, and your stroke should briefly pause at this end point to allow lymph to flow into the lymph nodes at the end of the channels.

Where swelling is very bad, massage the upper part of the limb first (knee to thigh) to clear these lymph channels before massaging the lower part (foot to knee). In cases where the whole limb is swollen through injury, effleurage may be given in elevation, with the leg supported on cushions and lifted to an angle of 20 to 30 degrees.

## Keypoint

When using a deep stroking massage (effleurage) to relieve swelling in the leg, massage the portion of the limb closest to the body (*proximal*) first to clear fluid from the lymphatic vessels. The tissue area further from the body (*distal*) is massaged second.

Where large body regions are covered, such as the posterior thigh or back, the skin is divided into regions to cover the whole area. With the posterior thigh, use strokes on the central (hamstring muscle), medial (adductor muscle) and lateral (abductor muscle) regions. With the back, contour the iliac crest (pelvis), then the centre (erector spinae muscle) and side of the back (latissimus dorsi muscle), and finally the shoulder (trapezius muscle) region (*see* figure 3.3).

## RHYTHM AND REPETITION

Aim for a natural rhythm, avoiding any sudden changes in pressure or timing. Perform 3–5 repetitions of the stroke on one part of the skin before moving onto another, aiming to cover the whole body area.

## PRESSURE

The pressure of effleurage may be varied from a light stroking action designed as a tactile (touch) stimulus only, to heavier pressure to move tissue fluid. Light fingertip pressure may be used to end a massage and maintain a feeling of relaxation – this type of stroking is called *brushing*. A slightly heavier technique which is still relaxing is poetically called *thousand hands* and involves drawing one hand across the body surface towards you (heel of the hand to fingers) and just as your fingertips are about to leave the skin, the heel of the other hand contacts the skin. The feeling is one of a continuous skin stimulation.

## 2. PETRISSAGE

The aim of petrissage movement is to encourage one area of tissue to move on another and so form an action called *tissue mobilisation* (*see* Keypoint box opposite). Petrissage covers *lifting* and *rolling* or *wringing* actions which are performed by lightly gripping (compressing) the skin and tissues and lifting them up. You should not use this technique where the skin is damaged or very thin. Lift with the whole of your hand, not just your fingertips, as this can pinch the skin painfully. As with all

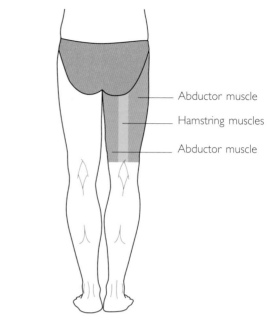

Abductor muscle

Hamstring muscles

Abductor muscle

(a) Posterior thigh

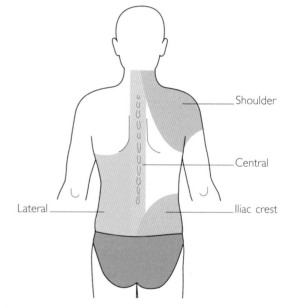

Shoulder

Central

Lateral

Iliac crest

(b) Back

**Figure 3.3** The skin is divided into areas to cover large regions of the body

massage techniques the power for the movement comes from your body and your hands simply transmit this power. With petrissage you will often find your body swaying with the action as you transfer your weight from one leg to the other, or from heel to toe, gently rocking your pelvis from side to side or forwards and backwards.

## Keypoint

Tissue mobilisation is performed when one section of tissue is moved on another. The effect is to encourage free movement of the tissue and may be used after injury or a heavy workout where waste products have built up in the tissues. The motion of the tissues encourages movement of tissue fluid and facilitates its reabsorption.

## TECHNIQUES

A wringing action (*see* figure 3.4) is performed by lifting the skin. Once lifted, move your hands forwards and backwards against each other to form an 'S' shape with the tissues. Release, move the hands to the next tissue section and repeat.

Rolling (*see* figure 3.5) lifts the skin without the underlying muscle. Now, the roll of skin may be moved by pressing the hands forwards across the skin surface so that the skin roll moves like a wave.

## RHYTHM AND REPETITION

Wringing can be performed fairly rapidly to stimulate blood flow, or more slowly allowing tissue to adapt. In the rolling action, the forward movement of the hands must be slow and sustained to allow the tissues time to respond and also to avoid skin pinching.

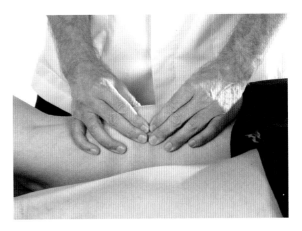

**Figure 3.4** Petrissage: a wringing action

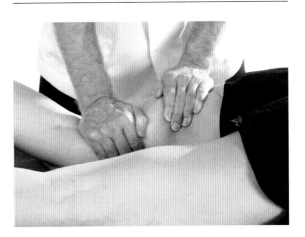

**Figure 3.5** Petrissage: a rolling action

## 3. TAPOTEMENT

Tapotement includes a variety of striking actions which are used to stimulate the tissues. The overlying skin becomes red as blood flows into the area, and nerve fibres are stimulated, which eases pain and stiffness. Striking actions are used over fleshy areas such as the back of the thigh, but not over bony areas such as the outside of the shin.

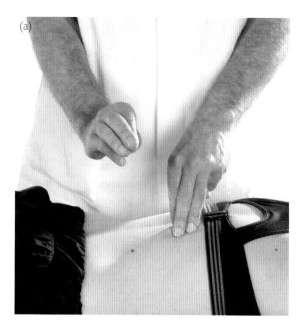

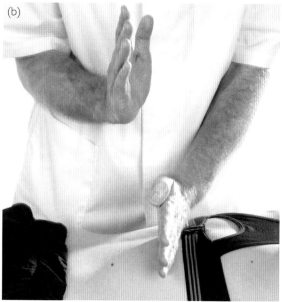

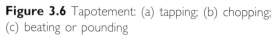

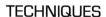

**Figure 3.6** Tapotement: (a) tapping; (b) chopping; (c) beating or pounding

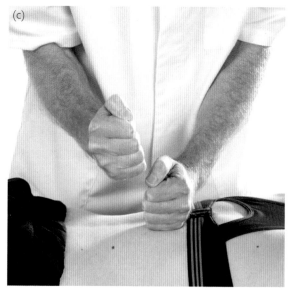

## TECHNIQUES

Strike the skin either with your fingertips (mild), which is known as *tapping*, the sides of your hands (heavier), which is known as *chopping*, or with the side of the open fist (intense), an action known as *beating* or *pounding* (*see* figure 3.6).

## RHYTHM AND REPETITIONS

Try to get a rhythm going slowly to begin with, but as you become more practiced you can speed up. The secret is to release your wrists so that your arms provide the power for the massage movement and your hands, being the massage tool, simply transmit the force that the arms have created.

## PRESSURE

As you move across the body, ease off the pressure as you approach thinner or more delicate regions to avoid causing pain or damaging the tissue. For example, if you are massaging the thigh, the striking action eases as you get close to the knee and is not performed at all over the kneecap (patella).

# 4. FRICTIONS

Frictional movements or 'frictions' are to and fro actions. Using a light touch the fingers move across the skin surface, but with a heavier touch the skin and finger moves as one unit, so it is the muscle beneath which receives the force of the massage. This deeper action is often performed across the fibres of a muscle or ligament and it is called a *deep transverse friction (DTF)* or *cross-fibre technique*. Frictions may also be performed in a circular fashion, a technique particularly useful on areas of dense swelling around a joint. For example, after an ankle sprain a pocket of firm swelling often remains below the outer ankle bone (lateral malleolus). Circular frictional massage may be used to break up the swelling and encourage the body to reabsorb it. Larger areas may be frictioned using the heels of your hands or the pisiform region of your inner wrist (*see* figure 3.7).

# 5. VIBRATION

Vibration may be used to stimulate the skin and underlying tissues, and is often used to change muscle tone, which is especially useful with neurological (nerve) conditions because it can help to stimulate nerves when they are conducting impulses poorly. Vibrations may also be used to work on a hollow body cavity, such as the lungs, and is often used in respiratory physiotherapy in hospitals as the vibration can loosen mucous secretions within the lungs so the patient can cough them out of the body.

## TECHNIQUES

The vibration may be performed by your hands or by using a massage machine. Tapotement techniques are used to strike the skin and can be

(a)

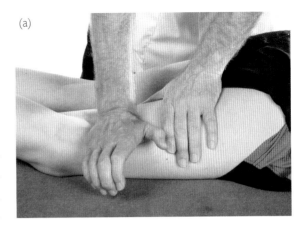

(b)

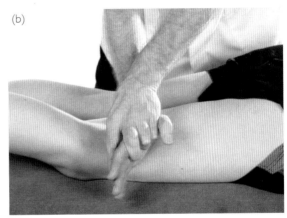

**Figure 3.7** Larger areas may be frictioned using: (a) the heels of your hands; (b) the pisiform region of your inner wrist

used rhythmically to induce vibration. Striking with the cupped hands (cupping) or the flexed fingers (flicking) are both examples of tapotement techniques which can be used rapidly to induce tissue vibration.

One of the most common vibration techniques in sports massage is to grip and lift the muscle (picking up) and then shake it. This may be performed on any long thick muscle (bipennate) such as the calf (gastrocnemius), arm (biceps and triceps), thigh (quadriceps and hamstrings) and top of the shoulder (upper trapezius). Shaking is often used to lower muscle tone and protective spasm prior to other massage techniques such as deep transverse frictions or joint mobilisation. The shaking action may desensitise the nerve (calm it down) thus reducing the number of electrical nerve impulses arriving at the muscle. Fewer nerve impulses can lead to a decrease in the muscle tone, therefore resulting in a softer, more pliable muscle.

A variety of mechanical massage machines are available (*see* figure 3.8). These generally produce different intensities of vibration. The contact area (head) of the machine usually comes in a variety of shapes and sizes to access large or small body areas. Although not as variable or specific as using

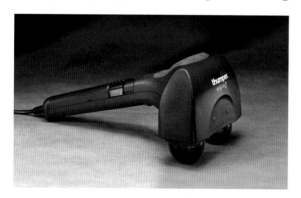

**Figure 3.8** A variety of mechanical massage machines are available

your own hands, a massage machine can be useful in cases where there is a large amount of swelling or where muscle spasm is intense. In each case the firm massage required will be very taxing on your hands, so to begin the massage using a machine can reduce your workload.

# ORDER OF TECHNIQUE APPLICATION

## ORDER OF MASSAGE TYPE

The order in which traditional massage techniques are applied is very much dependent on your client's needs. Generally is it best to begin and finish with effleurage movements as they ease your client into and out of the massage. The intensity of the massage movements builds, so light effleurage precedes more a more deeper action. Petrissage is next in terms of intensity, with wringing and rolling actions being used before tapotement techniques. Vibration and frictional techniques may be used either before or following tapotement. Where muscle tone is high, shaking may be used to relax muscle prior to petrissage. Where tone is lower, shaking and vibration may follow petrissage. Effleurage and light stroking are normally used to end a massage session. Table 3.1 lists a suggested order of technique application.

## ORDER IN WHICH TO MASSAGE THE BODY PARTS

Where full body massage is used it is normal to begin with your client face up and to target the face and neck, moving onto the shoulders and arms. The chest and ribs are then massaged and if abdominal massage is used this is given next.

| Table 3.1 | Suggested order of massage application |
|---|---|
| **Technique order** | **Body part order** |
| • Effleurage (light) | • Face |
| • Effleurage (deep) | • Neck and anterior shoulders |
| • Petrissage | • Right and left arms |
|   – Wringing | • Chest |
|   – Rolling | • Abdomen |
|   – Picking up | • Right thigh, shin and foot |
| • Tapotement | • Left foot, shin and thigh* |
|   – Cupping | • *Turn client* |
|   – Hacking | • Low back, mid-back, upper back |
|   – Beating | • Shoulders |
| • Shaking and vibration | • Neck and occiput (the posterior, or back, portion of the head) |
| • Frictions (local areas) | |
| • Effleurage (deep) | |
| • Effleurage (light) | |
| • Stroking | |

*Note: Where deep massage is used to improve lymph flow, the order is foot/shin/thigh for each leg.

Where massage is superficial, the front (anterior) aspect of one thigh is targeted, moving down to the shin and foot. Transfer to the other foot and work in the reverse order on the opposite leg, moving from the shin to anterior thigh. For deeper massage the direction changes so you work along the leg from foot (distal) to thigh (proximal), taking into account the direction of lymph flow.

The client then rolls onto their front, where the calf and posterior thigh of one leg is massaged followed by the calf and thigh of the other. The spine is next, moving from the lower (lumbar) spine to the thoracic, and finally the neck and posterior shoulders to finish.

The client is covered by towels or drapes placed on the chest, abdomen and legs. Each is removed while massage is applied and replaced to maintain body heat when the next section is massaged. As your client rolls over, to maintain modesty the central towel is held up in front of you as they roll onto their front, turning away from you.

As we shall see in the next chapter, clinical massage differs from traditional massage in the variety of techniques and the starting position. In addition, single body parts are commonly treated rather than the whole body.

# SPECIALIST MASSAGE TECHNIQUES

4

We have seen in chapter 3 that several traditional techniques are used in massage. These fall mainly into the category of Swedish massage and are often used for general (non-specific) care to target the whole body or limb where your client is in full health. For specific conditions where an injury has occurred or a clinical condition exists, more specialist techniques are often used, after whole body techniques have been given to allow the client to relax their tissues and for you to assess tissue tension.

In this chapter you will gain a general overview of the most commonly used specialist techniques. Although each technique is described separately, there is much overlap between techniques. Be prepared to change technique, depth and direction depending on your client's needs. In subsequent chapters you will see how these techniques can be put into practice on specific body parts.

## THE NATURE OF SOFT TISSUE

Basic human tissue begins in the foetus as a combination of three substances – cells, fibres and *ground substance* (matrix) forming into a generalised material called *connective tissue*. The proportion of each of these substances varies between tissues, but the basic structure remains much the same.

- The ground substance consists of fluid and proteins, which acts a bit like tissue 'glue'.
- The cells vary from tissue to tissue. In tendons and ligaments you have fibroblasts, in cartilage chondroblasts, and in bone osteoblasts. Each of these cells synthesises substances unique to their parent tissue; in the case of bone-forming osteoblasts, for example, one of the substances is calcium salts.
- There are two main types of fibre, collagen and elastin with additional *reticular* (cross-linking) fibres (*see* 'Definition' box) branching from the collagen. Collagen gives solidity while elastin, as the name suggests, gives elasticity.

### Definition

A reticular fibre is a specialist type of connective tissue which is able to form cross-links. By combining several fibres together in this way a meshwork is formed which acts as a supporting framework or scaffolding for other tissues to build on.

We are all familiar with bone, cartilage, ligaments, tendons and muscle. However, although it is convenient for us to name these as separate structures, they are not in fact separate at all.

## THE THREE LAYERS OF TISSUE

Our tissue begins its life from the moment of conception. As the cells which came together to form us divide, they form embryonic tissue which differentiates into three layers (germ layers): *ectoderm*, *mesoderm* and *endoderm*. The ectoderm eventually becomes skin and nerves, the endoderm forms the linings (*epithelium*) of your organs and glands and the mesoderm, quite literally, forms everything else. They are all interlinked.

## THE THREE TYPES OF FASCIA

All tissues are derived from connective tissue and their surfaces are continuous with each other. This continuous membrane covering is called *fascia* and we have three main types: superficial (under the skin), deep (around the muscles) and visceral (around the organs). These are joined in a network connecting every part of the body together. Like other tissues in the body, fascia has its own specialised cells, which it shares with tendons and ligaments, called fibroblasts.

## MYOFIBROBLASTS

Fascia also has offshoot cells called *myofibroblasts* and these can contract. Whereas a muscle receives a nerve impulse as a signal to cause instant shortening, myofibroblast contracts very slowly, taking up to 20 minutes to change their tension. The stimulation to change is not from a nerve impulse, but from a change in concentration of two important chemicals – histamine, released during inflammation, and oxytocin. Oxytocin is most commonly known as a female sex hormone but it has other important functions. It is a stress hormone and its concentration is changed during relaxation, stroking and pair bonding (*see* chapter 1). In other words, oxytocin is one of the most important hormones released during massage and its effect is directly on the tension of fascia.

### Keypoint

Changes in the chemical concentration of histamine released during inflammation, and oxytocin released during stroking have a direct effect on fascial tension.

Another feature of the fibroblast cells that is pertinent to massage is that they can respond to changes in tension within the fascia. Each cell has small protrusions, called integrins, on their surface. These stretch out at the front and loosen at the back meaning that the cell can pull itself along within the connective tissue ground substance. We can expect the fascia to respond to postural changes (altering tension and compression) by changing its structure, and these changes are not just local, but can run through the whole fascial layer. In turn fascia will also be affected by the tissue stress created by deep massage, so the very fabric of the tissues can change beneath your hands.

We know that general massage can affect the muscular system by relaxing it, the circulatory system by increasing blood flow, and the nervous system through sensation. The more specific massage techniques of this chapter will also affect these same systems, but in addition have a significant effect on connective tissue and fascia as well.

# FASCIAL RELEASE (FR)

Fascial release (also called *myofascial release* or *soft tissue release*) is a technique which targets the fascial network that travels throughout your body. With many of the massage techniques described in the previous chapter the emphasis was on gliding over the skin surface or lifting the tissues away from the bone. With FR, the technique is different.

There are two distinct phases of FR. Firstly you should use a sustained, fairly deep vertical pressure to sink into the target tissues. Once at the correct level, the direction of pressure changes, and you administer the second phase, which is to move the tissues more horizontally, pressing them in front of your fingers.

> **Keypoint**
>
> When performing facial release (FR), firstly sink into your client's tissues (depth) and then apply a horizontal force (shear) to lengthen the fascia.

This contrasts with skin rolling which is much more superficial, and consists of a horizontal pressure alone. Because you are no longer massaging along the skin, you need much less massage medium – sometimes a small amount of wax or thick massage cream is needed to protect your client's skin, but do not use so much that you slide over the skin surface.

## TECHNIQUES

Two main techniques are used in FR: *passive* and *active*. In each case the fascia should be fixed at one point (known as being locked) and stretched

> **Keypoint**
>
> It is essential that you are able to sustain the tissue lengthening action once you have sunk to the correct level. If you use too much of your massage medium and your fingers slide when they have sunk to the deeper tissue levels, the action can be very painful – a little like creating a 'Chinese burn' as a child.

at another. To lock the fascia, press into the deeper tissues, through the skin and subcutaneous fat, until you feel a resistance. If you go too far you will press into the muscle, and further still onto the bone.

Once you have pressed into the fascia, the FR lengthening may be applied by redirecting your fingers horizontally (known as *passive release, see* figure 4.1a) or asking your client to move their limb (known as *active release, see* figure 4.1b). For home use it is possible to instruct your client to perform both actions (lock and stretch) themselves, a technique sometimes termed *active-assisted* FR (*see* figure 4.1c).

## ENHANCING THE FR EFFECT THROUGH STRETCHING

The fascial techniques described above should aim to lengthen (stretch) the tissues. This effect can be enhanced by using a stretched limb position and then applying the massage technique. Gross stretching procedures, such as static stretch, dynamic stretch and PNF techniques are described in detail elsewhere (see *The Complete Guide to Stretching*, Norris 2010, published by A&C Black). The passive and active-assisted techniques used above may now be performed in a

(a)

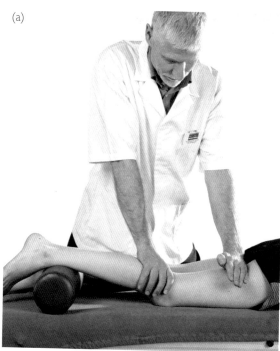

(b)

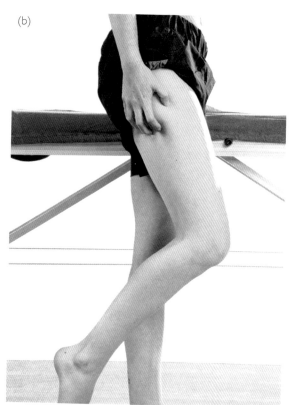

**Figure 4.1** Fascial release: (a) passive release; (b) active-assisted FR; (c) active release

(c)

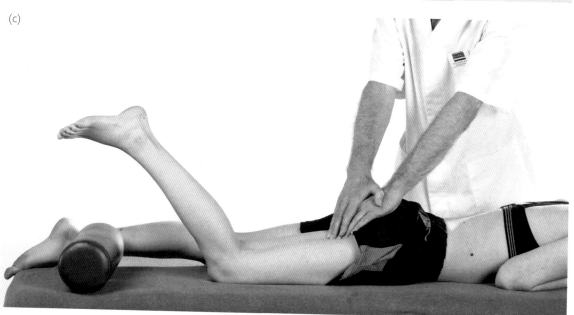

lengthened position. Use very little wax, aiming to dry stretch (tension) the skin and fascia. Hold the stretch for 20–30 seconds to allow a lengthways (longitudinal) reduction in tissue resistance so that the tissues give slightly.

## APPLYING A CROSSWAYS FORCE

This procedure can be further increased by applying a crossways (transverse) force to the tissues using a technique called *specific soft tissue mobilisation (SSTM)*. If we take a hamstring stretch as an example, traditionally we might use a straight leg

raise position with the client lying on their back (supine) to apply a passive longitudinal tension. To increase the tension on the tissue further, we can apply a transverse tension using SSTM in side lying. The client performs hip flexion (by moving the leg forwards and backwards) with their leg straight to lengthen their hamstrings (*see* figure 4.2a), and you then apply a passive transverse force into the hamstrings. The aim is to bend the muscle fibres over your fingers rather than to move your fingers over the fibres (*see* figure 4.2b) as would be the case in deep tissue massage, described below.

(a)

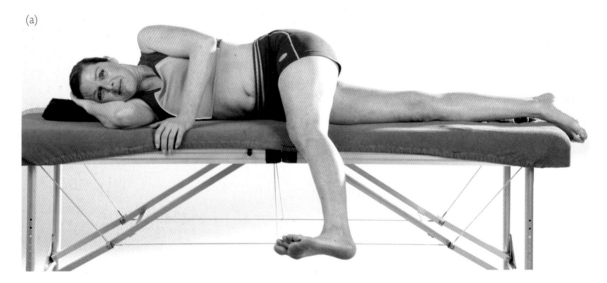

(b)

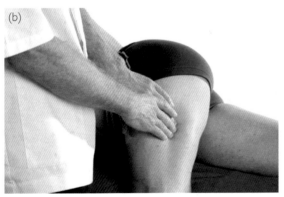

**Figure 4.2** Applying a crossways force: (a) the client performs hip flexion to lengthen the hamstrings; (b) the aim is to bend the muscle fibres over your fingers rather than to move your fingers over the fibres

# DEEP TISSUE MASSAGE (DTM)

The traditional Swedish massage techniques described in chapter 3 have a fairly superficial effect, targeting the skin and surface muscle. Sometimes it is necessary to use deeper techniques to work the more deeply placed muscles and other tissue. Deep tissue massage (DTM) focuses on two techniques of force application in particular: *compression* and *stretching*.

## COMPRESSION

Compression can be applied with a variety of contact areas. The smaller the contact area, the higher the compression value. This is the 'stiletto heel principle'; if you compare the impression made on a soft wooden floor between a heavy man in work boots and a lighter women in stilettos, the stiletto leaves a much deeper, but smaller, dent in the floor. This is because the weight is focused (distributed) in a much smaller area and this focused effect is very powerful. The amount of force you will impose on your client is proportional not just to how hard you press, but to the area of your surface contact.

> **Keypoint**
>
> In massage, compression force is proportional to (a) the surface area of your contact and (b) the amount of pressure you apply.

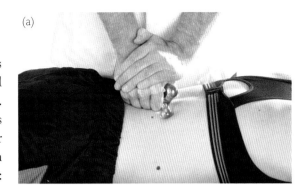

(a)

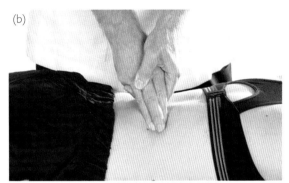

(b)

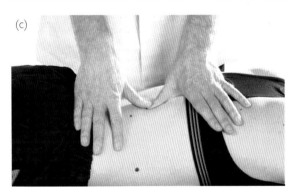

(c)

**Figure 4.3** Compression: (a) use a massage tool on a small contact area; (b) two or three fingers together to protect them; or (c) both thumbs

Using your fingertips or thumb pads will give you a smaller contact area, which will increase the amount of force you apply but will also place considerable stress on your fingers. Where a very small contact area is required, use a massage tool (*see* figure 4.3a) two or three fingers together to protect them (*see* figure 4.3b) or both thumbs (*see* figure 4.3c).

(a)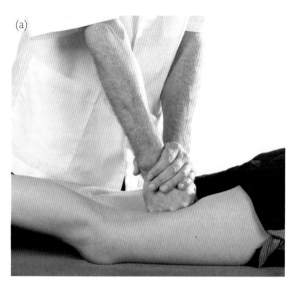

(b)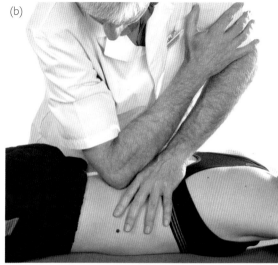

**Figure 4.4** Use your fist or elbow for larger areas

For a slightly larger contact area that still focuses the force powerfully, use your elbow. Larger still will be your fist or side of your forearm (*see* figure 4.4). The application of compression must be slow with a gradual build-up (crescendo). A rapidly applied force becomes a striking action, which when deep is very painful and will cause the muscles to tighten – exactly the reverse of what you require. Apply the compression force slowly, allowing the tissues to release. As they do so you will be able to judge how much more force is required and whether you should subtly alter the force direction to be more effective.

## STRETCHING

As with FR, stretching actions may be used to lengthen a whole region or to focus on a single tight area. Use very little massage medium to make sure you grip the skin rather than sliding over it. Often when working on a large area it is useful to use an X-grip or cross-hand grip (*see* figure 4.5), pressing evenly through the flat of your hands. The stretch should normally be maintained for 10–20 seconds to allow the tissues to elongate.

Tissue displays a property called *hyteresis* meaning that it will gradually give way or pay out under a constant force. If you stretch your tissues they will elongate. But if you continue to apply the same stretching force they will continue to elongate without the need for greater force. If you stretch rapidly or violently the tissues have a tendency to snap back at you. In other words, it is a case of stretch and wait, rather than stretch and force. Professional therapists often talk about waiting for the tissues to melt beneath their hands, and this analogy is absolutely correct because the ground substance of connective tissue changes from sol state (more solid) to a

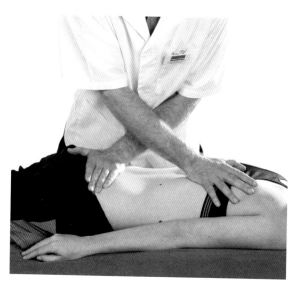

**Figure 4.5** Often when working on a large area it is useful to use an X-grip or cross-hand grip

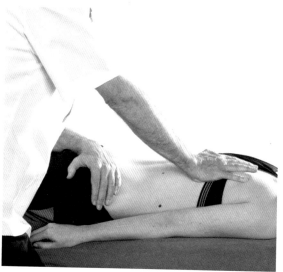

**Figure 4.6** Another method of applying stretch to the tissues is to use traction

gel state (more liquid) when force is applied to it and maintained.

Where local tissue stretching is required, one part of the tissue must be held still (locked) while the other portion is elongated (stretched), in much the same way as for FR. If we imagine a tight portion within a tissue as an elastic band with a knot in it, stretching the whole of the band (tissue) will not focus any greater stretch at the knot (tight region). Only by moving your hands closer to the knot will the stretch be focused

### Keypoint

Focus on the tightest part of the knot, giving it time to stretch.

more closely to that area. This is because tissue will always take the *path of least resistance*. Where part of a tissue is tighter and another part looser, when we stretch it is the looser area that gives out most. To focus the stretch to the tighter area, the looser area must be prevented from moving (i.e. locked). In this way the tighter area is given time to stretch.

### Traction

Another method of applying stretch to the tissues is to use traction. Here, rather than trying to increase the amount of joint movement (range of motion), you are trying to distract the tissues by pulling along the length of the limb as though you could pull the joint out of its socket. This imparts longitudinal tension to the tissues and feels very relieving to your client (*see* figure 4.6).

# TRIGGER POINT RELEASE (TRP)

When you massage a client you will often find areas of muscle which are tighter or seem to have a thicker consistency than others. Occasionally, however, rather than simply a thickening, you find a *tight band* or *nodule* which is very painful. As you press it the pain travels away (refers) from your fingers and the whole muscle reacts by suddenly jumping, causing your client to shout. This is a *trigger point (TrP)*. Trigger points (myofascial trigger points) are small areas of highly sensitive tissue lying within muscles especially. They normally present as either nodules, a little like a soft ball-bearing, or tight bands like soft short pencils. Sometimes clients will have identified these themselves because they are painful at rest. Sudden pressure or flicking your fingers across the TrP band can cause the muscle it is in to jump, a reaction known as the *twitch response* (jump sign). Some trigger points lie over traditional acupuncture points, while others are simply within the muscle. For this reason acupressure techniques (pressing over an acupuncture point) are often useful, and a major acupuncture point can serve as a starting point to finding a TrP through client palpation.

## ACTIVE AND LATENT TRP

A typical example of a trigger point is when it occurs in the upper trapezius muscle which has grown painful with prolonged sitting at the computer. At other times TrPs are painful only to your pressure, but they create the pain which your client may recognise as part of their condition. For example, clients with pain over the front of their shoulder may have a trigger point in the supraspinatus muscle at the top of their shoulder blade (scapula).

These two examples represent the most common types of TrP: *active* and *latent*. A latent TrP does not cause pain at rest, but only when it is palpated. An active TrP causes both pain and tenderness at rest or when the muscle is stretched during daily activities. Palpation of an active TrP causes pain and referral of the pain in a pattern, which mimics the patient's main symptoms.

> ## Keypoint
>
> TrPs are often found within the central belly of a muscle (a *central TrP*) or where the muscle attaches to the bone (*attachment TrP*). In the case of an attachment TrP, the TrP may be found both where muscle joins tendon (known as the *musculotendinous junction*) or where tendon joins bone (known as the *teno-osseous junction*).

> ## Keypoint
>
> TrPs are often noticeable during exercise and sport as they tend to restrict movement when the muscle they are in is stretched. For this reason they often have a relationship to posture and general body alignment. Tight muscle may cause an alteration in posture, but at the same time poor posture may cause tightness (muscle guarding).

## TECHNIQUES

We will look at three main techniques to release TrPs: *ischaemic compression*, *muscle stripping* and *positional release technique*.

## Ischaemic compression

With ischaemic compression, pressure is applied to the TrP slowly and built up progressively. The pressure is maintained until the local discomfort has reduced and the tissue changes from feeling hard to offering a softer resistance to your hands. Once the TrP has released, pause to allow your client to take a breath or two and then gently lengthen the muscle with a slow continuous stretch.

## Muscle stripping

The second technique, muscle stripping, is a deep stroking action a little like firm local effleurage (*see* page 38). Apply only enough massage medium to prevent friction, but allow firm grip to the tissues. Firm pressure is used all along the length of the taut band at a rate of approximately 2–3cm every 3 seconds. The direction should be from the hand or foot (distal) to the shoulder or hip (proximal) in order to create a type of milking action and cause an increase in local blood flow (known as *reflex hyperaemia*) that returns the muscle site to its normal condition.

## Positional release technique (PRT)

Positional release technique (PRT) is a method of relieving the pain created by a TrP. Instead of treating the TrP directly, it is used to assess or monitor the effect of body position. PRT seems to work by resetting the movement sense within the joints and soft tissues (known as *proprioception*) in some way, and by reducing pain by altering the level (threshold) at which pain is identified.

Having found a TrP, maintain the pressure over it while moving your client's limb (passively) to seek a *position of ease* (*see* Keypoint) – that is

### Keypoint

The position of ease is often one which takes the stretch off the muscle. For example, in the case of an upper trapezius muscle TrP, palpate it with your client in a seated position and then gently lift their shoulder blade in a shrugging action (elevation) and move their head sideways (known as *lateral flexion*) towards the side of pain. Shortening the muscle in this way takes the load away from it and allows the TrP to release.

the position which reduces the TrP sensation. Maintain this position of ease for 90–120 seconds and then repeat.

# DEEP TRANSVERSE FRICTION (DTF)

Deep transverse frictional massage (DTF) is a deep localised soft tissue technique often used by physiotherapists. It improves tissue function by increasing blood flow locally (known as *hyperaemia*) and reducing pain through the release of local chemicals.

DTF uses a crossways (transverse) sweeping action of the connective tissues which aims to discourage cross-link formation between collagen fibres, which can occur during healing. By applying oblique (shear) and lengthways (gliding) movements to the healing tissue, strength of the healing scar tissue may be improved and sticky adhesions reduced within the local area (*see* chapter 1).

Gentle DTF applied in the acute phase of healing stirs up the tissues just enough to stimulate healing but not so much that the healing process is disrupted. In the chronic stage of healing, DTF is said to soften and mobilise adhesions, sticky fibrils of connective tissue which form between the gliding surfaces of healing tissue and its surroundings, and is a useful adjunct to rehabilitation exercise.

## TECHNIQUE

DTF is performed with the client's skin and your fingers acting as a single unit. This is important because the aim is not to affect the skin, as with the friction techniques used in traditional Swedish massage, but to work the deeper tissues. A number of hand positions may be used to maximise the force applied to your client's tissues while at the same time minimising the stress imposed on your hands (*see* figure 4.7).

> **Keypoint**
>
> With DTF your fingers and the client's skin move as one unit. Do not glide over the skin surface as you are aiming to work the deeper tissues.

## USING DTF ON INJURED TISSUE

Because you are dealing with injured tissues, the point at which you apply DTF may not exactly correspond to your client's pain. Often pain is referred away (i.e. it appears in a location other than the area of perceived pain or injury) from the area of a lesion and it is important to target the precise location of the lesion rather than the pain.

DTF on tendons is generally given with the tendon in a stretched position, while muscles are treated in a relaxed position (known as *inner range*). Relaxing the muscle fibres in this way aids broadening and separation of the fibres to imitate normal function. Ligaments are placed under slight stretch to allow your fingers to reach the lesion and provide a firm base to work on.

> **Keypoint**
>
> Apply DTF to tendons with them stretched, and to muscles when they are relaxed. Ligaments are treated in a lengthened, but not fully stretched, position.

## ACUPRESSURE

We have seen that often TrPs correspond to acupuncture points. However, acupuncture points may be used to treat a body part to help stimulate healing even when they are not painful. Acupuncture is known as the use of thin needles placed within acupuncture points which lie on meridian pathways. In fact, acupuncture points may be treated with other forms of stimulation including local heat (known as moxibustion), vacuum suction (known as cupping), scrapping (known as guasha), electrical pulses (known as electroacupuncture) and finger pressure called tuina in Chinese medicine, shiatsu in Japanese medicine and acupressure in the West.

Modern research has found that many acupuncture points lie within regions of thickened fascia, and that these areas have very different properties than the surrounding tissues. Acupuncture points are more electrically active (they have a high conductivity and a low resistance) compared to the surrounding skin

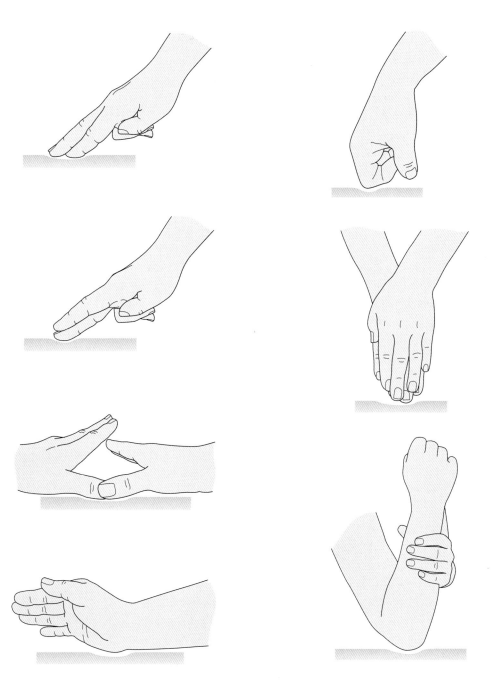

**Figure 4.7** In deep transverse friction a number of hand positions may be used to maximise the force applied to your client's tissues while at the same time minimising the stress imposed on your hands

and the meridian pathways themselves conduct electricity differently to the skin surrounding them. We know from research into the properties of fascia that the fascial network displays a form of biochemical signalling and it is likely that fascia is the area where the acupuncture effect is initiated.

## HOW DOES ACUPUNCTURE RELIEVE PAIN?

There has been much research into the way that acupuncture can relieve pain. Stimulation of acupuncture points produces pain chemicals (known as *opioids*) locally, and causes nerve signals to travel to the spinal cord to further enhance the pain response. From here signals go to the brain stem and up into areas of the brain responsible for hormone changes throughout the body (hypothalamus and pituitary glands) and changes in mood states (the limbic system).

## CHOOSING PRESSURE POINTS

Knowledge of the location of acupuncture points used in acupressure is helpful to the therapist using massage and a variety of point location guides are available (*see* Norris 2011). Sustained pressure is used over the acupuncture point for 30–120 seconds. The pressure is applied perpendicular to the skin surface. Points are selected close to the pain site and on the meridians passing through the area. Distal points on the meridians should also be used to enhance the effect.

## MUSCLE ENERGY TECHNIQUE (MET)

Muscle energy technique (MET) combines contraction of your client's muscle with a passive movement. The aim is to both alleviate pain and overcome movement limitation. The technique works on the same principle as PNF stretching (*see* page 48) where muscle is contracted against resistance (known as *isometric contraction*). Immediately following this contraction muscle tone reduces and stays slightly reduced for about 30 seconds. This period, called *post-isometric relaxation*, is used to achieve the clinical result. For example, if you were working on your client's hamstring muscles you could soften and lengthen them (reduce the muscle tone) by asking them to press their straight leg downwards against your resistance (hip extension) and then release it. The muscle tone will reduce slightly upon release, giving you the opportunity to gain further movement. The muscle reflexes involved in this technique are described in detail in C. M. Norris, *The Complete Guide to Stretching* 3rd edition (A&C Black, 2007), pages 53–60.

## TECHNIQUE

To apply MET you first need to identify a barrier to movement. To do this you move your client's body part to a position where stiffness or pain begins to occur. At this point you hold the body part still while your client contracts their muscles against your resistance (you try to move the body part, they try to stop you). The aim is to match their strength, but not to cause pain. The resistance you give (known as the *counter force*) should be just enough to prevent movement but not to cause pain. Hold the position for 10–20 seconds and then reassess the pain. If the pain has reduced but not gone completely, repeat the MET (*see* figure 4.9).

Where stiffness is a greater problem than pain (for example, as part of a subacute or chronic condition) MET may be used to increase the movement range. Now, after the period of muscle contraction, ask your client to move their limb into the stiff range while you follow the movement passively. Do not try to force the movement further, simply move within the free range and hold the end point to enable the tissue to release once more.

The relaxation phase of MET may be enhanced using the client's breath through a naturally occurring reflex (respiratory reflex). Ask them to breathe in slowly during contraction and out during relaxation. As your client exhales, encourage him or her to let go completely at the end of the movement. The breath is timed with the movement of the body part, but the breath should not be deep or held. Breathing too deeply or holding the breath can cause your client to become dizzy through hyperventilation.

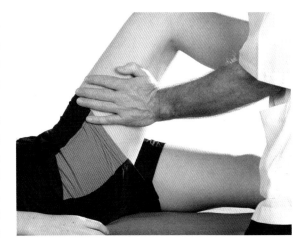

**Figure 4.8** Performing MET on a client

## Summary of key terms

- **Connective tissue** Generalised body material made up of cells, fibres and ground substance
- **Contact area** Area of client's skin which touches your finger/hand
- **Cross-link formation** Fibres formed between collagen fibres of injured tissue
- **Dynamic stretch** Stretching exercise involving movement
- **Epithelium** Lining of the organs and glands
- **Histamine** Chemical released during inflammation
- **Hypothalamus** Small area in the centre of the brain which releases hormones
- **Hysteresis** Property of tissue that enables it to give way or pay out under a constant force
- **Limbic system** Area at the lower back of the brain which controls emotions

- **Muscle guarding** Muscle tightness protecting a painful or injured body area
- **Opioid** Pain chemicals
- **Oxytocin** Female sex hormone also involved in the stress and relaxation response
- **Pathology** Medical or clinical condition affecting a client
- **Pituitary glands** Small pea-sized area in the brain connected to the hypothalamus which releases hormones
- **PNF stretch** Stretching exercise based on muscle reflexes
- **Static stretch** Stretching exercise which is held for 20–30 seconds
- **Twitch response** Reaction of a muscle to stimulation of a trigger point

# PLANNING THE TREATMENT // SESSION

5

Before we begin to use clinical massage we must determine our client's requirements. To use the same standard treatment techniques on all clients and each body part is both ineffective and in some cases very dangerous; there is no place for off-the-peg treatments in the clinical environment. Each client is different and each clinical condition is different, so our treatments must change accordingly.

We begin this chapter by looking at a methodical approach to deciding which treatments are appropriate, when they should be used and why. This process is called *clinical reasoning*.

## CLINICAL REASONING (CR)

The decisions we make during treatment with clinical massage should be based on a process of clinical reasoning (or clinical decision-making). Rather than applying standard treatments by using the same techniques with each client, we should assess our clients to determine their individual needs. Clinical reasoning (CR) is the thought process that we go through during the examination and application of clinical massage techniques. As therapists, we gather information from our clients and use this to develop an idea

> **Definition**
>
> In clinical reasoning a *hypothesis* is a theory which could explain our client's symptom behaviour.

(*hypothesis*, *see* 'Definition' box) about what could be wrong with them and what we should do to help them.

The process of CR involves interaction with our clients. When we do this we are really looking at them through a lens made up from our past knowledge and beliefs. Clearly the way that you look at a client as a qualified massage therapist will be very different to the way you would have looked at them before you entered this profession.

CR within massage therapy involves four essential components (*see* table 5.1).

CR entails collecting data (from signs and symptoms), analysing this data (making decisions) and then developing a treatment plan. It is important that you are able to justify why you are using a technique. What effect are you aiming for, and how will your clinical massage technique effect your client's condition?

| Table 5.1 | The four key components to clinical reasoning in massage |
|---|---|
| **Beliefs**<br>What are your beliefs about injury and healing, and how do these influence your treatment choices? | **Hypothesis**<br>What condition do you think explains your client's symptoms? |
| **Assessment**<br>What information do you get from the client prior to, during and after treatment? | **Expertise**<br>What clinical experience do you have of this particular condition? |

How do we gain this information? Essentially there are five ways in which clinical information is gained or influenced.

- 1. Source (where we think the client's symptoms are coming from)
- 2. Contributing factors (what makes their symptoms better or worse)
- 3. Precautions (what we should be cautious of when examining or treating)
- 4. Management (how we are going to treat them)
- 5. Prognosis (how we think they will react to our treatment)

## 1. SOURCE

As soon as your client walks into the room, you are *assessing* them. How they walk, talk and undress will all give clues. Contrast your view of someone who bounces into the room, bends over effortlessly to kick off their shoes and tells you they have just come back from a 5-mile run with someone who walks in slowly, showing pain on their face and unable to bend or reach forwards. The former client is less likely to have chronic low back pain than the latter. You have no proof of this of course, but your hypothesis is that because one client has unlimited movement and the other

reacts in a way that you have seen in those with back pain, it is likely that this particular patient may also have back pain. The essential feature here is that you have received information and compared it to your previous experience. Clearly, the experienced practitioner will be able to do this far better than a student, so the level of expertise that you have in relation to a clinical condition will influence your choice of treatment. Of course, you cannot choose to perform a massage technique on your client of which you are unaware.

> ### Keypoint
> Your expertise in relation to a clinical condition will influence your choice of treatment.

At the end of your assessment you have made a decision about the source of your client's symptoms (their back) and as you go through your assessment and gain further information you will support or disprove this hypothesis.

By continuing to gather information and compare it to what you think is wrong with your client you are using a process of *reviewing* your hypothesis. Sometimes the information may support your hypothesis. If you think your client has back pain when they come into the room, the fact that they experience pain when they bend to untie their shoes supports this. If they can bend freely and are able to get onto the bench easily, your original hypothesis of severe back pain may be incorrect.

### Keypoint

As treatment progresses, you gain further information from your client and apply the process of reflection to support, modify or refute your hypothesis.

## 2. CONTRIBUTING FACTORS

Contributing factors are those that aggravate your client's condition. These can sometimes be more important that the source of the problem itself. For example, the source of the problem may be your client's back muscles (the erector spinae) and the contributing factor is repeated bending at work. Unless you give your client advice about good back care and how to avoid bending from the back, their condition will not improve.

## 3. PRECAUTIONS

Precautions to examination and/or treatment are things that don't allow your client's condition to settle (repeated bending in the above example) or make it worse because they continue to stress the tissues, which increases pain and inflammation. It is especially important to identify anything which stirs your client's condition up so that you as the massage therapist can prevent making the condition worse by avoiding a certain type of massage action. If, for example, a client has an inflamed tendon that is made worse by mild movement, it would be unwise to use a vigorous massage technique. The fact that mild movement has made it worse would suggest that massage (a type of movement) if applied excessively may make their condition worse (we call this *symptom exacerbation*).

## 4. MANAGEMENT

The choice of management must consider if clinical massage is appropriate. It is easy to assume that because a client has come to see you, they need massage. It is important, however, to be able to say that massage is inappropriate should it be so at that particular stage and to refer the client to another healthcare or medical practitioner. If you consider that massage is appropriate you must now decide which techniques should be used and why (*justification of technique*). As you treat, you will continually gain feedback from your client – what they feel, how the tissues react to treatment and how they felt after treatment. These factors will give you an idea about the likely outcome following treatment (*prognosis*) and enable you to prepare your client for this.

## 5. PROGNOSIS

The prognosis you give is based on a number of factors. For example, is it likely that a client who has suffered from knee pain for six months will be pain free after a single treatment? They may expect to be, but your clinical experience with other patients and the nature of the healing process would suggest that several treatment sessions will be required. Remember also that clinical massage cannot cure everything. Clients will often put pressure on you to make them better, but in some cases a condition may be too serious or too far gone to help. If this is the case you must refer the client to another medical practitioner.

> **Keypoint**
>
> Be realistic about the likely outcome of treatment (prognosis).

## CLIENT EVALUATION

How do we gain information from our client to enable us to come up with a hypothesis to explain their complaint? This process is known as an assessment, or evaluation, and is most easily structured using the mnemonic SOAP, which is *subjective*, *objective*, *assessment* and *plan* (*see* figure 5.1).

### SOAP ASSESSMENT

The subjective assessment requires you to question your client and/or take a history. Clinical conditions often have a definite pattern, for example an acute injury (one which happens suddenly) would normally develop from the patient having a history of injury in that particular region, while a chronic injury (one developing slowly) will usually have resulted from overuse of a body part during a regular or daily activity. During the subjective assessment we aim to identify these patterns. To do this we should ask questions in a variety of categories and, as a guide, figure 5.2 shows typical categories used by physiotherapists.

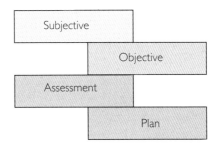

**Figure 5.1** The SOAP chart is helpful for assessing your client's needs

| **Category** |
|---|
| Age and occupation |
| Site and spread |
| Onset and duration |
| Symptoms and behaviour |
| Medical considerations |

**Figure 5.2** These are the typical categories you should question during the subjective assessment

#### Age and occupation

Asking questions about age is important because certain conditions, such as osteoarthritis, can be more common in older clients. It also crucial to establish the occupation of your client as low back pain can occur in anyone, but manual workers have very different stresses imposed on the spine to desk-bound individuals, for example. In addition the advice for aftercare will obviously vary, so gaining a wider knowledge of the typical activities which a client is returning to is important.

#### Site and spread of symptoms

The site and spread of symptoms (something a client may complain of) can give clues to pain referral. For example, a disc injury in the low back may trap the sciatic nerve sending pain into the leg (known as *sciatica*), and this particular client may complain of leg pain but be unaware that they have a back condition. Equally, pain can be referred from a condition even when a nerve is not trapped. For example, a frozen shoulder may often give a deep gnawing pain which travels across the front of the shoulder and into the upper arm. Failure to identify this could lead to treatment of the wrong tissues, which is to say that you could end up targeting the arm rather than the shoulder itself, which is where the problem originates.

### Onset and duration of symptoms

Asking questions regarding the onset and duration of symptoms will clarify the difference between a sudden onset (acute) condition and one which has developed slowly over time (overuse). This information will help you to identify the stage of the injury and its healing and the likely condition of the injured tissues.

### Symptoms and behaviour

Learning more about key symptoms and their behaviour will provide you with information regarding any issues that may make the client's condition better or worse. For example, a chronic stiff joint is typically better for gentle mobilising exercise while an acute joint normally reacts to exercise with increasing pain as the condition is stirred up and you would need to avoid this in your treatment plan.

### Medical considerations

A medical history should be taken as it is crucial to know if a client has medical conditions other than the injury they are presenting with and if they are taking any medications for that condition which may affect or be affected by massage. A simple medical questionnaire should be filled in prior to treatment, and you should question your client more closely on areas which are likely to be affected by massage. Questionnaires of this type are often available through therapists' governing bodies and you should use these examples or contact your training college for a suitable document. Always liaise with your client's GP to ensure that your treatment does not conflict with treatments being given by other practitioners.

## REACTION TO TREATMENT

Once you have given clinical massage, your next treatment session begins with a reassessment of your client's symptoms. Have they improved or worsened? How did your client react to the treatment? The simple mnemonic SIN, which is severity, irritability and nature, can be helpful here. Clinically we combine our impression of these three factors to limit treatment where SIN factors are high.

### Severity

The severity of a condition can be determined by the amount of pain the client is in. In hospitals, this is typically measured using a pain scale (visual analogue scale or VAS) from 1 to 10, 1 representing little pain and 10 representing maximum pain. You should ask your patient to decide where they fall on this scale. This is easier to record for assessment and more is a more informative method than the patient simply saying that their condition is 'painful' and is 'getting better' following treatment.

### Irritability

Irritability is how quickly a condition is 'stirred up', generally measured as the length of time your client does something before their pain increases (walking, bending, lifting, for example) and how quickly the pain settles once the activity is stopped. If your client has an injured knee which is painful after only two or three steps and it takes 2 minutes to settle, it is more irritable than someone with a similar condition who can walk for 10 minutes before pain occurs, and then it settles within a couple of seconds.

## Nature

The nature of a condition reflects the stage of healing, whether acute, subacute or chronic. Also important is the type of injury – traumatic or overuse – and the amount of tissue damage – large (for example extensive bruising to the hamstrings) or small (for example a minor calf tear).

# CHOOSING APPROPRIATE TECHNIQUES

There are dozens of clinical massage techniques that we will cover in chapters 6–9, so how do you know which ones to use? To decide we need to look at the aims of the treatment. What do you hope to achieve by using clinical massage? It may be that you want to reduce pain, relax muscle, aid venous return (the rate of blood flow back to the heart), increase lymphatic draining, mobilise soft tissue or all of these. The most important questions to ask are what treatment and recovery is realistic and what should be applied first.

In general, begin with traditional massage techniques to relax your client and allow your hands to get used to their tissues. In fact, this portion of the treatment forms part of your clinical assessment as you are assessing *selective tissue tension* – literally getting to know their

body and where the tissues are most and least tense, for example. Use effleurage and petrissage movements with a slow flowing motion.

Next, decide on the level of pain. If the level is high (above 6 on a VAS scale) your techniques must be light and brief. Where pain is low (under 4) you may use deeper techniques for longer periods. Your aim should be to reduce pain or at least not exacerbate the pain.

Of the techniques that are described in chapter 4 both trigger point release (TrP release) and acupressure are used mostly to target pain. If you detect a nodule or tight band in a muscle and deep palpation (touching) reproduces your client's pain, use TrP release. Where no tissue changes are apparent, but pain is very high, select light general massage techniques followed by acupressure. Muscle energy techniques (MET) may also be used as they focus on muscle as the source of pain.

Deeper tissue techniques such as deep transverse frictions (DTF), deep tissue massage (DTM) and fascial release (FR) are used predominantly where tight tissue rather than pain is the primary problem. Again, begin with general massage techniques to become familiar with the tissues and then go deeper. The byword here is progression. Gradually increase the force of your massage technique as the tissue tension reduces. This is a little like gym training where to continue to strengthen muscle by adding more weight (muscle overload) must be used. Now, however, it is tissue overload beneath your hands which is changing. Finish the technique with some relaxing massage techniques to reduce post-treatment soreness, but warn your client that their tissues are likely to be sore for 24–48 hours following treatment.

# PROGRESSING TREATMENT

At the beginning of each follow-up session you should assess your client once again. Reassessment will not be as long as your initial assessment, but will focus on significant findings and items which your treatment aimed to change. For example, you may measure pain and daily pattern of symptoms, range of motion and functional changes such as time-to-pain onset (the time it takes for the pain to present). The aim of reassessment at the beginning of a treatment session is to judge whether you should simply repeat your treatment using the same clinical massage techniques or if you need to change them. Where post-treatment soreness was very marked you may decide to use lighter techniques or to use deep techniques for a shorter period, for example. Where tissue tightness was reduced without significant post-treatment soreness you may increase the depth of a specific technique or the length of time for which it is applied.

### Keypoint

Remember that clinical massage is only one aspect of treatment. Build in self-care, home exercise or self-treatment techniques, such as trigger point pressure massage, between treatment sessions so that the client can maintain the clinical effect of your treatment.

# OUTCOME MEASURES

An outcome measure is really a standard against which treatment results can be measured. How do we know that a clinical massage treatment has been effective? We need to measure something before, perhaps during, and certainly after the treatment to track our client's changes. Outcome measures may include:

- the number of painkillers that a client is taking (if this reduces it would indicate that pain is lessening);
- the length of walking distance with a knee injury;
- lifting capacity with a back injury.

# REASSESSMENT DOCUMENTS

The key here is that the outcome measure has to be relevant to the client. It is no good saying that pain has reduced and so the client is discharged if the client's main concern is their knee giving way, which has not changed. For this reason we normally use a patient reported outcome measure (PROM). These are normally standard hospital forms which measure changes in mobility, self-care, usual activities, pain and anxiety, for example.

To really be specific to what is important to your client you may choose to let them define what they want measured and then allow them to measure it. The standard hospital test to do this is a measure yourself medical outcome profile (MYMOP) (Paterson 1996). This questionnaire asks your client to define two symptoms which affect them (bother them) most, one activity which is important to them and then to rate their general feeling of well-being during the last week. The MYMOP form is available as a free download from http://sites.pcmd.ac.uk/mymop/files/MYMOP_questionnaire_initial_form.pdf.

You may feel that you do not need to be this specific if, for example, you are working with a client purely for relaxation purposes. However, it is important to measure and record outcomes so you can review your work in the future. In addition, as part of good record-keeping, the outcome you achieved should be recorded on your client's records together with full details of any home care advice.

# CONSENT

Prior to carrying out clinical massage it is essential to gain your client's consent. It is a fundamental principle in the free world that all individuals have the right to determine what happens to their own body, so much so, that touching your client without gaining consent may constitute the legal charge of *battery* (*see* 'Definition' box), or even sexual assault.

> ## Definition
>
> *Battery* is defined in law as an intentional unpermitted act causing harmful or offensive contact with the 'person' of another.

Quite apart from the legal ramifications, explaining what you intend to do before you carry out a clinical massage procedure is courteous and helps to create a relationship of trust. Essentially, consent demonstrates that the risks, benefits and outcomes of your clinical massage treatment have been explained to your client and they have made their own decision about treatment.

For consent to be appropriate (valid) there are three requirements:

- 1. Your client must have the capacity to consent, they must be *competent*.
- 2. Their consent must be *voluntary*.

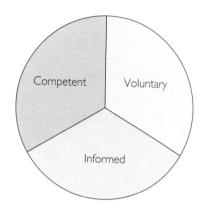

**Figure 5.3** Requirements of consent

- 3. Sufficient *information* must have been given for them to make an informed decision about their treatment.

## 1. COMPETENT CONSENT

Clients over the age of 18 are considered competent to give consent, while younger clients may still consent, but an adult should witness this. To ensure that your client is competent, ask yourself if they can understand the information that you are giving them. Secondly, are they in a fit state to make a decision? If they are in a lot of pain, for example, they may agree to anything which they think will reduce their pain without necessarily thinking about it. Use this period to explain your treatment to your client and get them to participate in their recovery. Remember that clients bring with them their own belief system, and you should respect this.

## 2. VOLUNTARY CONSENT

Make sure that you do not pressure your client into giving consent. Their consent must be voluntary. This is especially important with the elderly or where your client does not speak the same language. It is easy to skate over the consent process assuming that they have understood your explanation of treatment when they have not.

Remember also that you as a professional can easily be intimidating to a patient, and they may not feel comfortable about saying 'no' when they would really wish to. Make sure you are as approachable as possible and avoid appearing 'superior' to your client.

## 3. INFORMED CONSENT

Consent must be informed. You should explain what the clinical massage treatment is going to achieve (the outcome) as well as any risks, such as soreness following treatment, skin discolouration or minor local swelling (weal). Remember also that you need to keep your client informed as you change your treatment techniques, and that they have a right to withdraw their consent at any time.

## WRITTEN, VERBAL AND IMPLIED CONSENT

Although many clinics have written consent forms, which in legal terms are said to show *evidence of process*, it is important that you as a therapist also gain consent from your client. A receptionist, for example, may not be able to inform your client of likely treatment outcomes or risks, so although a form can be used as part of the consent process you should still raise the question of consent in addition to seeing the form. Perhaps go through the form with the client, drawing their attention to items which you can elaborate on.

Your treatment records should record that consent was obtained, and how this was obtained. Consent may be either *explicit* (written or verbal) or *implied*. Implied consent means that you client, for example, held out their limb for you to examine it (*see* 'Definition' box). However, asking specifically if it is OK for you to touch an area and recording this in your treatment notes is important for sensitive areas, for example, around the breast or genitals in the case of chest or groin injury.

### Definition

In legal terms *implied consent* is that which is inferred from signs and actions, or by inaction or silence.

### Summary of key terms

- **Clinical reasoning (CR)** Describes the thought process that a therapist goes through during the examination and application of clinical massage techniques
- **Contributing factors** Factors that make the client's condition worse
- **Explicit consent** Written or verbal consent
- **Implied consent** Where the patient holds out their arm or similar for you to examine
- **Mobilising exercise** Exercise given to ease stiffness in a joint
- **Selective tissue tension** Examining tissues by stressing to different degrees

# LOWER LIMB TECHNIQUES

**6**

## ANATOMY REFRESHER

The lower limb consists of the pelvis, thigh bone (femur) and two shinbones (tibia and fibula) some of which you are able to touch (palpate), as detailed in table 6.1.

| Table 6.1 | Palpable structures in the lower limb |
| --- | --- |
| **Anatomical structure** | **Common name** |
| Iliac crest | Rim of pelvis |
| Femur | Thigh bone |
| Tibia | Inner shinbone |
| Fibula | Outer shinbone |
| Anterior or posterior superior iliac spine (ASIS/PSIS) | Sharp point at front of pelvis |
| Greater trochanter | Knobble on side of hip |
| Ischial tuberosity | Sitting bone |
| Lateral epicondyle | Raised area above outside of knee joint |
| Medial epicondyle | Raised area above inside of knee joint |
| Patella | Kneecap |
| Tibial tuberosity | Bump below the kneecap |
| Tibial crest | Sharp rim of shinbone |
| Lateral malleolus | Outer ankle bone |
| Medial malleolus | Inner ankle bone |
| Calcaneus | Heel bone |
| Tubercle of navicular | Highest point of inner foot arch |

## BONE STRUCTURES IN THE LOWER LIMB

At the front of the outer pelvis is the anterior superior iliac spine (ASIS) which forms the attachment of the strap-like sartorius muscle passing diagonally across the front of the thigh to the inner knee. The ASIS is quite sharp and on very thin clients you may need to put a folded towel or pad beneath it when your client is lying on their front. At the side of the hip is the greater trochanter, an area which is covered by a balloon-like, fluid-filled sac called a *bursa*, which provides a cushion between bones and tendons and/or muscles around a joint. The bursa can swell if someone falls onto their hip, which is a common injury in skiing. Your sitting bone is the ischial tuberosity which forms the upper attachment of the hamstring muscles at the back of your thigh. At the side of the knee, just above the joint, are two raised areas. On the outside of the knee this is the lateral epicondyle and on the inside the medial epicondyle, each forming the base of attachment for the outer knee ligaments (collateral ligaments). The shinbones are covered by muscle except for the bump beneath the kneecap, the tibial tuberosity, which forms the attachment of the patellar tendon, and the sharp front edge of the shin, the tibial crest.

The ankle bones (lateral and medial malleolus) form the attachments of the ankle ligaments which are commonly sprained in sport. The heel actually consists of two bones, the talus, forming the mortise within the ankle joint, and the heel bone proper, the calcaneus. The highest point on the inner arch of the foot (medial longitudinal arch) is the navicular bone which forms the keystone to the arch. These palpable areas, which are easily touched during massage, are often referred to as *bony landmarks* (*see* figure 6.1).

## MUSCLE STRUCTURES IN THE LOWER LIMB

The front of the thigh is made up of the quadriceps, a group of four muscles which straighten (extend) your knee. One of this group, the rectus femoris, straightens your knee but also bends (flexes) your hip. It is the kicking muscle and is commonly injured with mistimed violent kicking actions. The back of the thigh consists of the hamstring group, attaching from your sitting bone to the top of your shin (tibia). These muscles bend your knee but also extend your hip, so are involved in running actions. They are commonly pulled and often need clinical massage.

The inner thigh muscles (adductors) travel from the inner rib of your pelvis to the inside top of your thigh bone. The outer thigh muscles (abductors) come from your outer pelvis to the outside of your knee (femur, tibia and fibula). The abductor muscles (gluteals and tensor fascia lata) attach into the iliotibial band (ITB) which forms the shallow groove down the outside of your leg along the trouser seam. This structure is often very tight in sport and can often require clinical massage treatment.

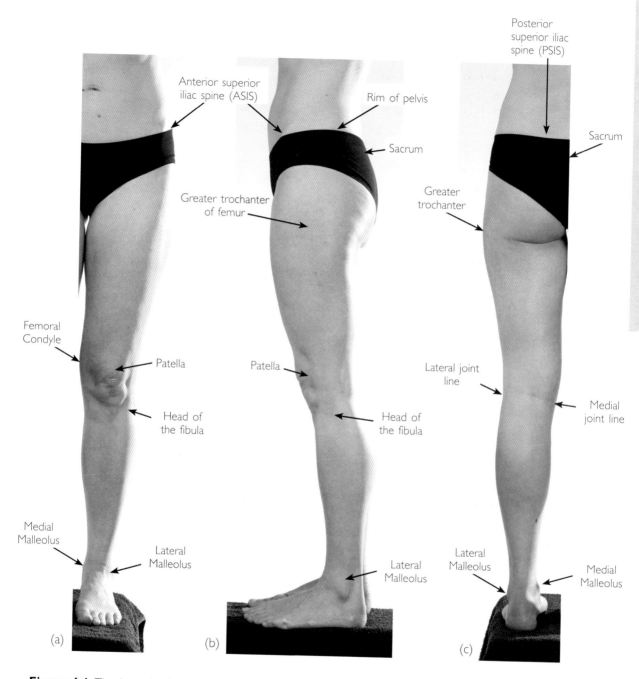

**Figure 6.1** The bony landmarks of the lower limb: (a) front; (b) side; (c) back

## Exercise 6.1 Hamstring muscle belly, effleurage

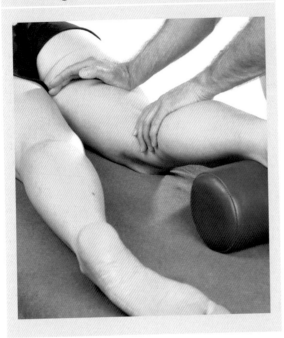

### Purpose

To relax hamstring muscle tightness or spasm and increase local blood flow to the muscles.

### Preparation

Begin with your client lying on their front with a cushion or block beneath their skin to flex the knee and relax the hamstrings slightly. Use the outside (little finger side) of your far hand, supported by your near hand as a broad massage contact.

### Action

Target the hamstrings in three strips – lateral, central and medial – providing an even sweeping pressure along their full length from the back of the knee to the buttock. Release tension when you reach the buttock and slide the hand back to the knee maintaining skin contact on the downward stroke. Repeat the action three times on each strip and continue until the required effect is achieved.

### Tips

Apply less pressure over the knee where the muscles are tendinous and increase pressure towards the middle and top of the stroke where the muscle thickens.

### Points to note

The downwards stroke maintains skin contact, but not pressure so that the pressure emphasis is distal to proximal in the direction of lymph flow. Ensure that the downwards stroke is not so light that you tickle your client, however, as the back of the thigh is very sensitive in some individuals.

**Exercise 6.2** Hamstring muscle belly, vibration

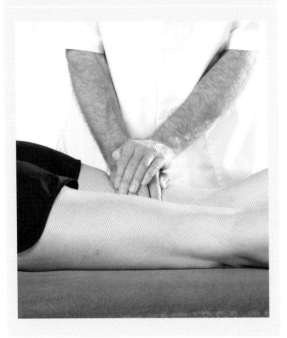

## Purpose
To change tone in the hamstring muscles and increase local blood flow.

## Preparation
Begin with your client lying on their front with a cushion or block beneath their skin to flex the knee and relax the hamstrings slightly. Use one cupped hand (palm down) alone or supported by the other to increase force. Stand side on to your client with your hand perpendicular to their posterior thigh so that your hand and forearm form a straight line.

## Action
Press down onto the hamstrings to increase contact force and vibrate (shake) the muscle using a rapid but small (high velocity, low amplitude) forward and backward motion of your hand and forearm.

## Tips
Ensure that your hand maintains contact with the posterior thigh and does not slide across the skin.

## Points to note
Vibrating a muscle may either increase or reduce muscle tone depending on the resting tone of the muscle. Where tone is low (hypotonic), vibration may stimulate muscle contraction and where tone is high (hypertonic), vibration can reduce tone.

**Exercise 6.3** Hamstring insertion, DTF with hip flexed

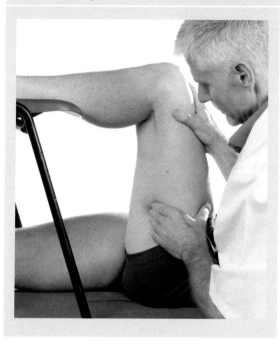

## Purpose

To target the hamstring insertion onto the sitting bone (ischial tuberosity) using deep transverse frictions (DTF).

## Preparation

Begin with your client lying on their back with their affected leg bent at the hip and knee, calf resting on a stool. Sit close to their bent leg. Press your index finger and middle finger together and bend them slightly to create your massage contact.

## Action

Press into the muscle attachment at the sitting bone and perform a DTF action, sweeping across the muscle fibres. The amount of movement will only be about 5–10cm. Make sure that your fingers stay in contact with your client's skin rather than gliding over it.

## Tips

To maintain sufficient pressure on your client's tissue, brace your elbow against your own body. Apply pressure as you draw your hand towards yourself and release the pressure as you return your hand. Alternating pressure in this way allows your hand time to recover between strokes.

## Points to note

This starting position relaxes the hamstrings at the knee but stretches them at the hip. You can vary the starting position by moving the stool closer to (greater hip flexion) or further away from your client (less hip flexion).

## Purpose

To target the hamstring insertion onto the sitting bone (ischial tuberosity) using deep tissue massage (DTM).

## Preparation

Begin with your client lying on their front. Place a towel beneath their kneecap and allow their feet to drop over the bench end.

## Action

Use your elbow as the massage contact. Place the point of your elbow onto the upper portion of the hamstrings as they move onto the sitting bone. Use the webspace of your other hand to lock your elbow into place and prevent it slipping over your client's skin. Gradually press into the area, hold the tension for 1–2 seconds and then release. Move along the whole upper portion of the hamstrings, in total about 15–20cm in length and 5–10cm in width.

## Tips

Vary the intensity and direction of your pressure as the tissue will be more tense as you get closer to the sitting bone. If you find the pressure from your elbow difficult to control, substitute the knuckles of your index and middle fingers pressed together.

**Exercise 6.4** Hamstring insertion, DTM prone lying

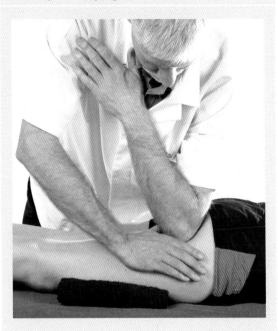

## Points to note

Normally when massaging a client on their front you would place a roll beneath their shins. This allows the knee to unlock and takes stress from the back of the knee (known as *popliteal structures*). However, this position also relaxes the hamstrings slightly. By allowing your client's feet to drop over the bench end the leg is fully extended and the hamstrings place on minimal stretch. Pressure over the kneecap is reduced by placing a towel beneath their knee.

**Exercise 6.5** Hamstring upper portion, DTM with stretch

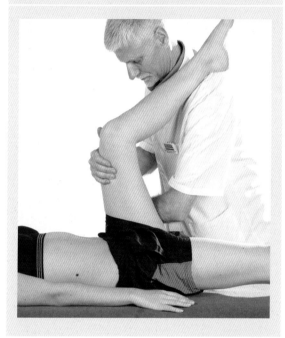

## Purpose

To apply deep tissue massage (DTM) during active stretching.

## Preparation

Begin with your client lying on their back with their affected (for example, left) leg close to the bench edge. Stand (stride standing) with your left leg nearest the bench edge and your right leg forwards. Place your client's calf onto your left shoulder (protect your shoulder with a folded towel). Use the edge of your left forearm as your massage contact.

## Action

Firstly press into your client's hamstring muscle while fixing their leg with your right hand. Initially apply pressure inwards and upwards towards their buttock to stretch the fascia. Repeat this action for 2–3 minutes until the tissues feel less resistant. Secondly, press into their posterior thigh and keep your forearm still as they lift their calf up from your shoulder (leg extension) and then rest it down again. Perform 5–10 repetitions of this action, allowing their hamstring muscles to glide beneath your forearm.

## Tips

If you find balancing hard while performing this technique, use a perching position where you place your left buttock on the edge of the bench.

## Points to note

As you support your client's leg with your right hand make sure you do not press directly over their kneecap, as this can be painful.

## Exercise 6.6 Hamstring, MET

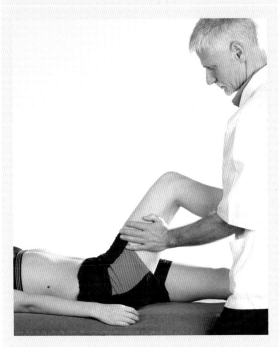

### Purpose
To manage spasm and shortening of the hamstring muscles using muscle energy technique (MET).

### Preparation
Begin with your client lying on their back (supine) with their affected leg closer to you. Grasp their leg at the ankle with your near hand and their thigh with your far hand, keeping their leg bent (flexed) at both the knee and hip.

### Action
Keeping their knee slightly bent, move your client's leg to the onset of resistance (barrier) or pain. Ask them to bend their knee against your resistance and hold the contracted position for 10–20 seconds. As they release, move the leg upwards to the new movement barrier.

### Tips
Contraction force should be 20–50 per cent of maximum. The lower value is applied in painful conditions, the higher where tightness exists alone. With an athlete, place their calf on your shoulder to provide a more stable resistance.

### Points to note
Bending the knee more relaxes the hamstrings slightly at the knee and therefore targets the upper portion of the muscle.

**Exercise 6.7** Posterior thigh fascial stretch

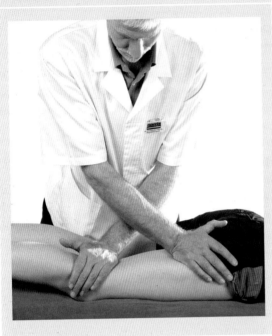

## Purpose

To stretch the superficial fascia of the posterior thigh from the knee to the buttock.

## Preparation

Begin with your client lying on their front with a folded towel beneath their calf.

## Action

Use a cross-hand grip (X-grip) to stretch the skin and fascia, placing your left hand flat on the upper leg and your right hand flat on the lower leg. Without allowing your hands to slide over the skin surface, lean forwards slightly, pressing your weight into your hands.

## Tips

If you find taking weight through your wrists stressful on this area, use a forearm contact instead. When using your forearms do not cross your hands. Fix with one flat hand and apply skin traction with the side of your other forearm.

## Points to note

The action should be to press your hands apart to stretch the thigh area between your hands. You will need to reposition your hands several times to cover the whole of the posterior thigh.

**Exercise 6.8** Hamstring belly, DTF

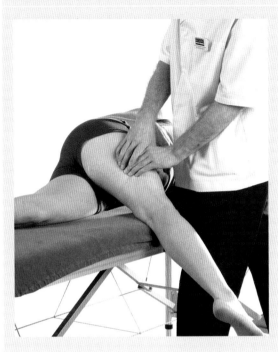

### Purpose

To apply deep transverse friction (DTF) massage to the hamstring muscle bellies.

### Preparation

Begin with your client lying on their side facing you, with their hip flexed to 90 degrees. Your massage contact for this technique is one hand supported by the other. Your fingers are flexed, wrist locked straight.

### Action

Keeping your fingers flexed but locked, grasp the centre of the hamstring muscle bellies and draw your hands across the muscle fibres without sliding over the skin.

### Tips

The power for this action comes from body sway rather than movement of your fingers or wrists. Apply power on the upwards stroke but release power on the downwards stroke.

### Points to note

If you find your hands begin to ache with this action you are using your hands too much. Remember that your hands are the tools which transmit rather than create force. The force must come from body sway, and your fingers simply direct this force onto the hamstring muscle bellies.

**Exercise 6.9** Inner knee joint line, FR

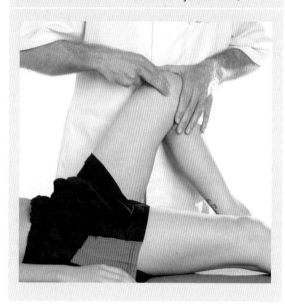

## Purpose

To release the fascia and deep ligament (coronary ligament) of the knee using fascial release (FR).

## Preparation

Begin with your client sitting with their knee bent to 90 degrees and foot turned outwards (lateral tibial rotation). Your massage contact is your index and middle fingers held together and bent slightly, supported by your other hand.

## Action

Place your fingers onto your client's knee joint line, which is a shallow groove approximately level with the bottom of the kneecap. Sweep your fingers forwards and backwards in a line covering 3–5cm.

## Tips

If you find it difficult to use your fingers in this way substitute your thumbs instead.

## Points to note

The action of turning the foot outwards twists the shinbone laterally, tightening the tissues on the inner aspect of the knee. This action brings the tissues you are targeting closer to the surface and to your fingers.

## Exercise **6.10** DTF to medial collateral ligament of knee

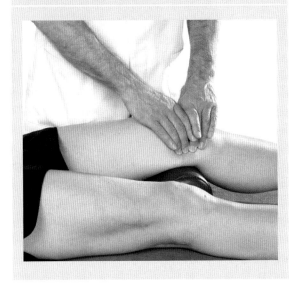

### Tips
Following MCL injury the knee may be stiff due to adhesions. The aim of the DTF is to reduce the adherence of adhesions and increase the range of motion. Use comfortable full range starting positions, but do not force the movement range.

### Points to note
The deep fibres of the MCL blend with the joint capsule while the more superficial fibres move more freely as the joint bends, and the fibres tighten at different movement ranges. You need to target both sets of fibres, hence DTF is given in both knee flexed and extended positions. Note also that there is a bursa beneath the front of the ligament, just below the joint line (*see* figure 6.2).

### Purpose
To target the deep and superficial fibres of the medical collateral ligament (MCL) of the knee during the subacute phase of injury using deep transverse friction (DTF).

### Preparation
Begin with the patients lying or sitting the legs straight (long sitting). The injured knee is supported on a pillow so that it lies just short of full extension.

### Action
Impart DTF firstly with the knee in full comfortable extension and then full comfortable flexion. During extension the movement is directed vertically and in flexion diagonally, in line with the joint surface. Begin the action lightly and increase depth as the client's pain reduces.

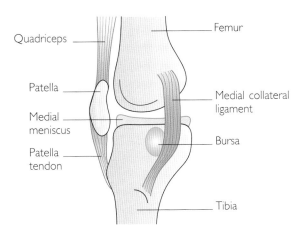

**Figure 6.2** There is a bursa beneath the front of the medial collateral ligament in the knee, just below the joint line

81

## Exercise 6.11 Kneecap FR

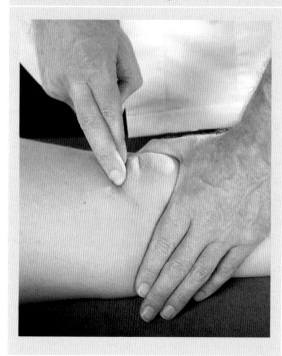

### Purpose

To release the fascial tissues attaching to the kneecap, using fascial release (FR).

### Preparation

Begin with your patient sitting with their leg straight. Encourage them to relax their thigh muscles by having them tense and relax their thigh two to three times. Use your index finger supported by your middle finger as your massage contact.

### Action

Place your two fingers just above your client's kneecap. Use your other hands (lightly cupped) to tip the kneecap from the base so that the top is lifted away from the thigh bone slightly. Keep your fingers tight together and your wrist locked and perform the soft tissue release by turning your forearm up and down (pronation and supination), and pressing your forearm forwards and backwards.

### Tips

If you find using your fingers difficult, use the knife edge of your hand on the little finger side. If any old swelling is present around the kneecap, begin by using traditional circular frictions prior to using more specialist techniques. Do use deep massage if fresh swelling is present.

### Points to note

You may target the tissues below or to the sides of the patella equally. In each case, tip the kneecap slightly upwards at the point closest to your hand. In this way the tissues beneath your fingers are tightened to create a firmer base to work on.

## Exercise 6.12 Patellar tendon, DTF

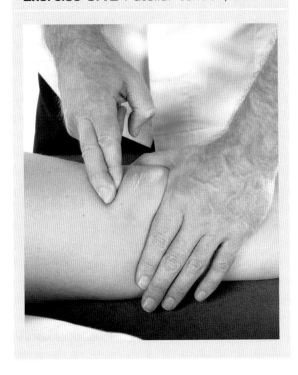

### Purpose
To target the patellar tendon attachments either above or below the kneecap using deep transverse friction (DTF).

### Preparation
Begin with your client sitting with their leg straight. Use quadriceps vibrations to relax the quads so that the patella is easily movable. Locate the position of pain in the area either below (infrapatellar) or above (suprapatellar) the patella. Use one hand to stabilise the patella and produce the DTF action with the other hand using the side of the forefinger supported by the rest of the hand, fingers straight.

### Action
To administer DTF to the suprapatellar region stand side on to your client and use your left hand to gently press the patella upwards (superiorly). Use the side of the index finger of your right hand to impart the DTF using a transverse action (across the leg). To administer DTF to the infrapatellar region, use your right hand to gently press the patella downwards (inferiorly) while imparting the DTF with the index finger of your left hand.

### Tips
Where pain occurs close to the bone (teno-osseous junction) the patella may be tipped upwards allowing your index finger to press slightly beneath the patella. The action is the same, but can also include a scooping movement using pronation and supination of your forearm.

### Points to note
Movement of the patella can be tender initially, so general massage using circular friction massage around the patella and effleurage to the quadriceps may also be used as a precursor to DTF.

**Exercise 6.13** DTM around patellar rim

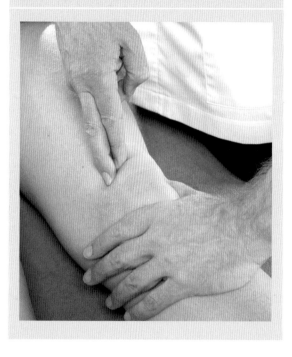

## Action

Apply circular frictions around the whole rim of the patella. Focus greater pressure above the patella (suprapatellar pouch) and to the sides of the patella tendon (infrapatellar fat pads), as shown in figure 6.3.

## Tips

Use a minimum amount of massage cream to reduce skin friction but to maintain skin contact in order to apply sufficient force. The longer the swelling has been present, the thicker it will be, so the greater amount of force will be required.

## Points to note

Where swelling has filled the suprapatellar pouch it will have spread throughout the whole knee joint, so the knee may be unable to straighten fully.

## Purpose

To reduce swelling around the patella using deep tissue massage (DTM).

## Preparation

Begin with your client sitting on a bench with their leg straight, resting on a pillow or cushion. Use your index finger supported by either your middle finger alone (two-finger contact) or middle and fourth fingers (three-finger contact) as your massage tool.

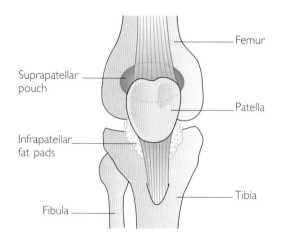

**Figure 6.3** Focus pressure on the patella (suprapatellar pouch) and to the sides of the patella tendon (infrapatellar fat pads)

## Exercise 6.14 Posterior thigh acupressure

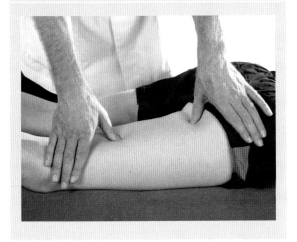

### Action
Use your thumbs or two/three fingers pressed together to compress each acupuncture point. Press perpendicular to the skin and hold the pressure for 20–30 seconds.

### Tips
In cases where pain is intense, rather than use direct pressure an electrical pulse stimulator pen may be substituted.

### Points to note
Use deeper pressure on fleshy points (BL-36/BL-37/BL-57) and lighter pressure where the tissues beneath are more delicate (BL-40/BL-60).

### Purpose
Using acupressure to reduce posterior thigh pain.

### Preparation
Acupuncture points on the posterior thigh lie on the bladder (BL) meridian. Most commonly used are BL-36 in the centre of the buttock fold, close to the ischial tuberosity, BL-40 close to the centre of the posterior knee joint line (popliteal crease), directly between the tendons of biceps femoris and semitendinosus, and BL-37 just above the midpoint of the meridian line running between BL-36 and BL-40. BL-57 may also be used, lying midway between the knee and ankle joints at the midpoint of the two gastrocnemius bellies, and BL-60 on the outside of the ankle midway between the lateral malleolus and the Achilles tendon may be used where pain spreads down the leg beyond the knee (*see* figure 6.4).

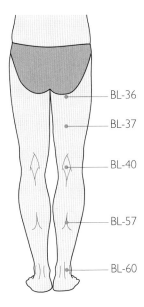

**Figure 6.4** This shows the acupuncture points on the posterior thigh

## Exercise 6.15 Upper ITB FR

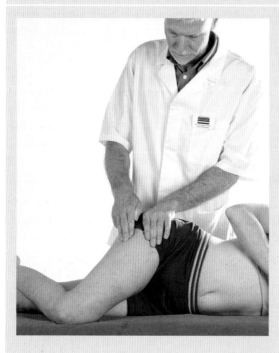

### Purpose

To release fascia tension in the upper portion of the ilio tibial band (ITB) using fascial release (FR).

### Preparation

Your client should lie on their side with their affected leg on top. Their knee is bent to 90 degrees with the side of their knee resting on the treatment bench. Fix their leg with your left hand (keeping it flat) and use the edge of your right forearm as your massage contact.

### Action

Apply deep massage to the ITB from the greater trochanter downwards (*see* table 6.1). Also address the tensor fascia lata (TFL) muscle in front of the trochanter and the front portion of the gluteus maximus behind. Search out trigger points in both muscles. For the TFL the trigger point is often found midway between the trochanter and the iliac crest and for the gluteus maximus in the space between the trochanter and the sacrum.

### Tips

It is sometimes more comfortable for you to sit (perch) on the bench below your client's knee.

### Points to note

If your client has a very tight ITB, this position may be uncomfortable. If so, begin with their knee supported on a folded towel or block (yoga block). As the ITB tension releases you may find their knee lowers and you no longer need the block.

## Exercise **6.16** Lower ITB FR

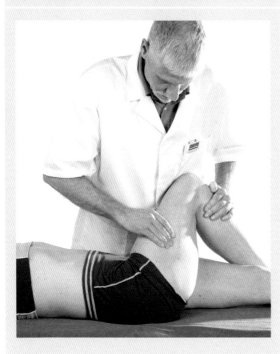

### Purpose

To release fascia tension in the lower portion of the ilio tibial band (ITB) using fascial release (FR).

### Preparation

Have your client lie on their back and bend their unaffected left leg. Move their affected right leg across the bench into adduction and cross their left leg over it. Stand to your client's left side.

### Action

Use the curved fingers on one hand drawn into a solid ridge, supported by your other hand. Reach across your client's leg and apply deep transverse frictions (DTF) and specific soft tissue mobilisation (SSTM). To administer DTF draw your hands towards you (upwards and across the body) to contour the leg. To administer SSTM hook your fingers beneath the ITB and draw it towards you, bending the fascia. Hold the stretched position for 30–60 seconds.

### Tips

If you find this position uncomfortable for SSTM, use the side lying position of upper ITB release. To access the lower ITB use the little finger side (pisiform grip) of your hand.

### Points to note

The ITB is a thick and tough structure so work into it gradually. It may take 3–4 minutes before your notice any change in tissue tension.

## Exercise 6.17 ITB/TFL combined MET

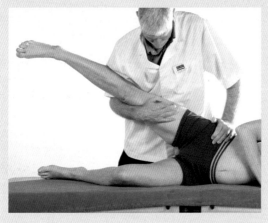

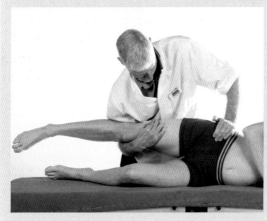

### Purpose

To reduce tone in the tensor fascia lata (TFL) muscle and lengthen the ilio tibial band (ITB) at the side of the thigh using muscle energy technique (MET).

### Preparation

Begin with your client lying on their unaffected side. Stand behind them, place your right hand over the rim of their pelvis and support their affected leg using your left arm, looping your forearm beneath it.

### Action

Abduct and extend their affected leg and press down onto their pelvis to prevent any pelvis tilt. From this position gradually lower their leg into adduction while maintaining slight (5–10 degree) hip extension. When you reach the maximum comfortable range, ask your client to try to lift their leg against your resistance (known as *isometric hip abduction*). Maintain this contraction for 5–10 seconds and then repeat the stretch.

### Tips

Press down onto the pelvis only with enough force to prevent pelvic tilt. Too much pressure can be painful over the bony pelvic rim.

### Points to note

Flexing your client's knee will increase the effect of the stretch on the lower portion of the ITB and draw the ITB behind the tibial epicondyle. In cases of ITB friction syndrome at the knee this method is often more clinically effective.

## Exercise **6.18** Abductor muscle acupressure

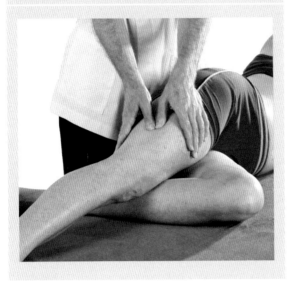

### Purpose

To reduce pain from abductor muscle tightness using acupressure.

### Preparation

Begin with your client in side lying with their lower leg bent and upper leg dropped into adduction. The gallbladder (GB) acupuncture meridian is targeted. GB-29 lies between the greater trochanter and the anterior superior iliac spine (ASIS) within the gluteus medius muscle on the outside of the hip. GB-31 is just over two hand widths above the outer (lateral) knee joint line within the ITB. GB-34, one finger width down and in from the top of the outer shinbone (head of the fibula) and GB-40, one finger width down and in from the outer ankle bone (lateral malleolus) are used as points away from the pain but on the gallbladder meridian (*see* figure 6.5).

### Action

Use your thumbs or two/three fingers pressed together to compress each acupuncture point. Press perpendicular to the skin and hold the pressure for 20–30 seconds.

### Tips

In cases where pain is intense, rather than administer direct pressure, use an electrical pulse stimulator pen.

### Points to note

Use deeper pressure on fleshy points (GB-29/ GB-31) and lighter pressure where the tissues beneath are more delicate (GB-34/GB-40). Tightness in the ITB is often reduced using this technique, but this reduction must be maintained by giving your client stretches for the area. See *The Complete Guide to Stretching*, 3rd edition (Norris 2007), pages 109–10 for details of abductor stretching exercises.

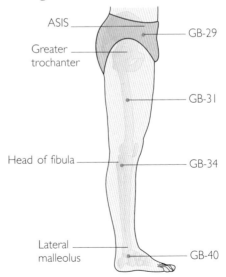

**Figure 6.5** Targeting the gall bladder acupuncture meridian

## Exercise 6.19 Upper insertion adductor muscle, DTF

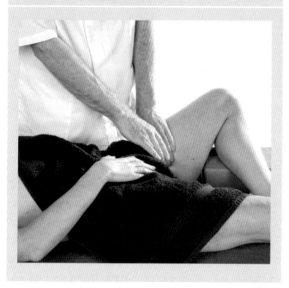

### Purpose

To target the upper portion of the adductor muscles (especially adductor longus) following adductor muscle strain using deep transverse friction (DTF).

### Preparation

Begin with your client lying with their affected leg bent and turned outwards (hip flexed, abducted and externally rotated). Their knee should rest on a pillow for support and a folded towel is used to cover their groin for privacy.

### Action

Apply the DTF action using the pads of your semi-flexed fingers, pressed together in a single unit. Target the most painful portion of the muscle which may be the junction between the muscle and tendon (musculotendinous junction) 3–5cm below the pubis, the tendon itself above this point, or the point of tendon attachment to the pubic bone (teno-osseous junction). Press your finger pads firmly into your client's skin and maintain skin contact as you impart the frictional form to the tendon tissue beneath. Use a broad (3–4cm) sweep to take in the whole tendon mass.

### Tips

Where the teno-osseous junction is affected in males, ask your client to draw their testicles to the side away from your working hand.

### Points to note

Strain of the adductor muscle at its attachment to the pubic bone must be distinguished from osteitis pubis which is an inflammation of the pubic symphasis joint. When in doubt you should refer your client to their GP or physiotherapist as an X-ray may be required which can show rarefied (less dense) bone. For details see *Managing Sports Injuries* (Norris 2011), pages 151–2.

## Exercise 6.20 Adductor muscle, MET

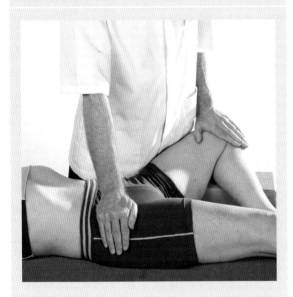

### Purpose
To reduce tone in the adductor muscles prior to stretching using muscle energy technique (MET).

### Preparation
Begin with your client lying with their affected leg bent and turned outwards (hip flexed, abducted and externally rotated). Their knee should rest on a stack of folded towels for support.

### Action
For your client's right leg, place your left hand on the left rim of their pelvis to prevent it lifting from the bench. Place the flat of your right hand over the inside of your client's knee. Ask them to attempt to lift their knee off the folded towels (adduction), against your resistance. Hold the tension (known as *isometric muscle contraction*) for 10 seconds and then release. Reduce the number of towels so the range of motion to adduction is increased, and repeat three times.

### Tips
Because the length of your client's femur provides a long lever, you do not need to press down hard. Use enough pressure to have your client press upwards with about 30–50 per cent of their maximum.

### Points to note
If your client has very tight adductor muscles, their leg will rest higher. Your action now will be to pull their inner knee towards you rather than press it down to the bench.

**Exercise 6.21** Quadriceps, DTM using compression

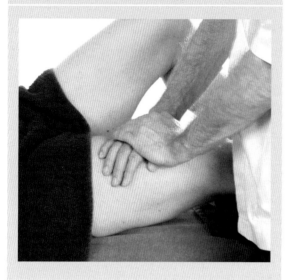

## Purpose

To give deep tissue massage (DTM) to the quadriceps muscle.

## Preparation

Have your client lie on their back with a folded towel beneath their knee

## Action

Compress the quadriceps muscles with the flat of your fist reinforced by your other hand. Rock your body forwards to generate the compression force, hold for 4–5 seconds and then release. Move your hand further up the muscle and repeat.

## Tips

Compression with your fist is easier at the sides of the quadriceps. If you find the action awkward over the top of the muscles, use your forearm, but be cautious not to use the sharp side of your forearm (ulna bone) – use the fleshier portion towards your elbow.

## Points to note

Compression over the quadriceps can be painful as you can sandwich the muscles between your fist and the thigh bone beneath. Using a broader contact area reduces the risk of the technique being painful.

### Exercise 6.22 Adductor release using DTM in frog position

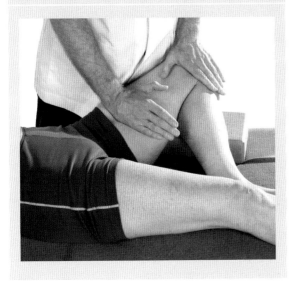

### Purpose

To release tension in the adductor muscles using deep tissue massage (DTM).

### Preparation

Begin with your client lying on their back with their affected leg closest to you. Bend their knee to 90 degrees and place their foot against the knee of the straight leg. Rest the knee of their affected leg onto your waist.

### Action

Stabilise your client's leg with one hand and use the edge of your other forearm to apply firstly compression and then effleurage to the adductor muscles, from the knee to the groin.

### Tips

As tension releases in the adductor muscles, allow your client's knee to rest lower on your waist.

### Points to note

The adductor muscles attach right up into the groin onto the pubic bone. Massaging in this area is very intimate but it is necessary, to reach the whole of the muscle. Seek your client's permission before doing this and protect their privacy using a towel to cover their groin area. They may place their own hand over their genitals.

**Exercise 6.23** Pes anserine, FR

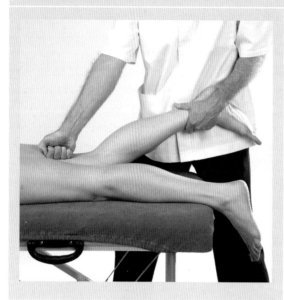

## Purpose

To target the pes anserine structures (sartorius, gracilis and semitendinosus tendons) on the upper inner portion of the shinbone using fascial release (FR).

## Preparation

Begin with your client lying on their front with their knees slightly apart, feet over the end of the bench. Bend their affected knee to 90 degree and allow their foot to move outwards twisting their thigh bone (medial rotation of the femur).

## Action

Apply a tissue lock using the flat of your fist onto the lower medial portion of the hamstrings and adductors. Maintaining this lock, use your other hand to guide your client's leg into extension, imparting a stretch to the fascia on the lower medial portion of the knee.

## Tips

If your client finds their kneecap is pressing into the bench surface, place a folded towel beneath their lower thigh just short of their kneecap.

## Points to note

In case of pes anserine pain, begin by palpating the area to assess pain intensity. Perform the fascial release and then retest the area. If the technique is successful your client's pain should reduce.

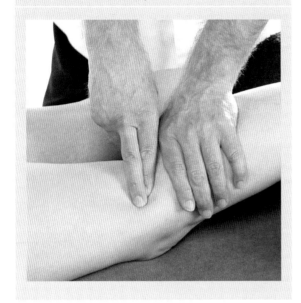

**Exercise 6.24** Popliteus, TrP release

### Purpose
To reduce pain and spasm when locking the knee using trigger point (TrP) release.

### Preparation
Begin with your client lying on their front with a folded towel beneath their thigh and their foot over the bench end. Locate the trigger point approximately two thumb widths below and one thumb width medial to the centre of the knee crease.

### Action
Use fingertip compression to target the TrP. Increase pressure gradually and hold the compression for 30–120 seconds, until pain subsides.

### Tips
The posterior aspect of the knee is delicate, so less pressure is required over this point than with other TrPs.

### Points to note
The popliteus muscle is often a key element to knee pain occurring as the knee is locked out straight. Popliteus acts to unlock the knee by rotating the femur on the tibia when the foot is on the ground. The rotation movement of the bones (known as the *screw home effect*) twists the knee and locks the joint out in the final few degrees of extension. If the popliteus is in spasm or is painful following hyperextension injury, the knee often unlocks with a sudden give rather than a normal controlled motion.

**Exercise 6.25** Calf compression in hook lying, DTM

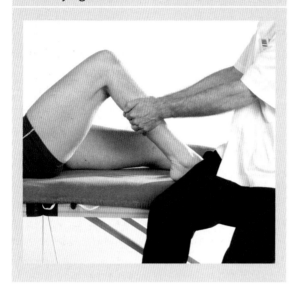

### Purpose

To apply deep tissue massage (DTM) to the gastrocnemius muscle.

### Preparation

Begin with your client lying on their back with their knees bent and foot flat on the bench. Perch on the bench and place your whole curved hands behind their calf.

### Action

Keeping your hands behind your client's calf, lean back slightly, compressing the calf muscle towards the bone. Alternate your hands, working along the whole length of the calf.

### Tips

If you find your client's foot slides on the bench, place a folded towel over their foot and sit on their toes lightly.

### Points to note

For stronger compression, interlock your fingers and use both hands together.

**Exercise 6.26** Calf muscle vibration

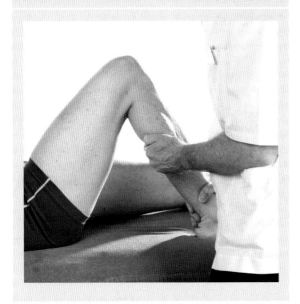

## Purpose
To relax the calf muscles prior to stretching or deep tissue massage (DTM).

## Preparation
Begin with your client lying on a bench with their knees bent and feet flat. To treat the near leg, use your left hand on their shin to prevent their foot from slipping. Your right hand is your massage contact – use it slightly cupped to support the calf muscle bulk.

## Action
Keep a straight line through your wrist and forearm and use a rapid but rhythmic forwards and backwards action to vibrate the calf from side to side.

## Tips
Begin using slow movements to allow your client to get used to the action and then speed up. A sudden rapid onset of shaking can cause muscle tone to increase rather than reduce.

## Points to note
The weight of the calf pulls the muscle down and away from the bone in this starting position.

**Exercise 6.27** Gastrocnemius TrP release

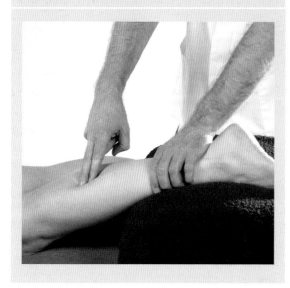

## Purpose

To reduce pain and muscle spasm in the gastrocnemius muscle using trigger point (TrP) release.

## Preparation

Begin with your client lying on their front with their knee bent, shin supported on a roll (bolster) or several folded towels. You massage contact is two knuckles pressed together to reinforce them.

## Action

Locate the TrP of each muscle belly, approximately 1–1.5 hand breadths below the centre of the knee crease. The lateral belly is found on the outside and the medial belly on the inside of the calf. Compress the area using gradually increasing pressure (crescendo) and hold the compression for 30–120 seconds.

## Tips

Follow the procedure with a passive calf stretch, straightening your client's leg and pressing their foot upwards (known as *ankle dorsiflexion*). Hold the stretch for 20–30 seconds.

## Points to note

Encourage your client to breathe normally, there is a tendency for them to hold their breath when a technique is slightly painful.

**Exercise 6.28** Gastrocnemius muscle, DTF

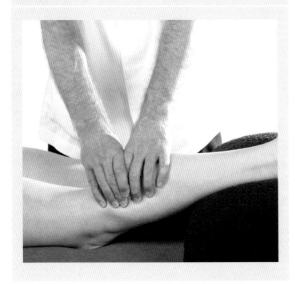

### Purpose
To target the gastrocnemius muscle using deep transverse friction (DTF) to broaden the muscles fibres.

### Preparation
Begin with your client lying on their front with their knee bent and supported on pillows or the inclined bench end. Use your finger pads of one hand supported by the other as your massage contact.

### Action
Press you fingers into your client's skin to prevent them slipping, and impart the DTF using a smooth to and fro action.

### Tips
Keep your elbows tucked into your sides and create the force of the action using the sway of your body. Your hands transmit rather than create the massage force.

### Points to note
Follow the treatment by giving your client light exercise to contract (broaden) and then lightly stretch (lengthen) the muscle fibres.

**Exercise 6.29** Anterior tibial release, DTM

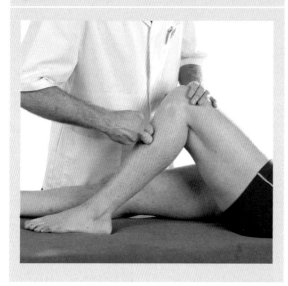

## Purpose

To reduce pain from shin splints (known as *anterior tibial syndrome*) using deep tissue massage (DTM).

## Preparation

Begin with your client sitting with their leg bent to 90 degrees, their foot flat on the bench. Fold your index and middle finger of your right hand at the end joints only. Keep the large knuckle joint (metacarpal phalangeal joint) straight and reinforce your fingers with your thumb.

## Action

Stabilise your client's leg with your left hand and use your right hand knuckles to press into the tibialis anterior muscle on the outside of the shin.

## Tips

To press harder, straighten your client's leg and press with the knuckles of your right hand, supported and guided by your left hand.

## Points to note

The tibialis anterior muscle is thicker towards the knee and its trigger point is located approximately 1.5 hand widths below the knee joint line to the outside of the sharp crest of the tibia bone.

**Exercise 6.30** Peroneal DTM

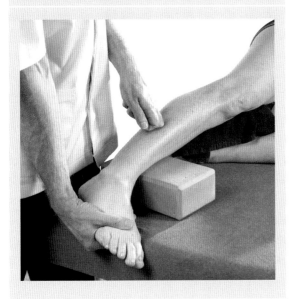

## Purpose

To reduce pain over the lower outer shin (lateral compartment syndrome) using deep tissue massage (DTM).

## Preparation

Begin with your client lying on their side with their foot over the bench end and relaxed into inward (inverted) position. Fold your index and middle finger of your right hand at the end joints only. Keep the large knuckle joint (metacarpal phalangeal joint) straight and reinforce your fingers with your thumb.

## Action

Stabilise your client's leg with your left hand and use your right-hand knuckles to press into the peroneus muscles on the lower outer portion of the shin.

## Tips

To work deeper, draw your client's foot down and inwards (plantarflexion and inversion) with one hand to place the peronei muscles on stretch. Press with the knuckles of your other hand while maintaining the stretch.

## Points to note

To turn this technique into an active soft tissue release (STR), hold your knuckles still and ask your client to pull their foot up and out (eversion and dorsiflexion) and then to relax and repeat the action. The peronei muscles will slide beneath your palpating knuckles.

**Exercise 6.31** Peroneal muscle, MET

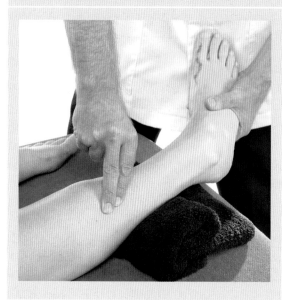

## Purpose

To release tension in the peroneal muscles on the outside of the shin using muscle energy technique (MET).

## Preparation

Begin with your client lying with their foot over the bench end, or calf on a block to allow the heel to move freely. Stand at the end of the bench and, if you are treating the left leg, stabilise your client's shin with your left hand. Grasp their foot with your thumb to their sole (plantar surface) and fingers on top of the foot (dorsum), knuckles to the outside (lateral aspect).

## Action

Draw your client's foot inwards (inversion) so that the sole of the foot faces to the midline of the body. Hold this position and then ask your client to push their foot outwards (eversion) against your resistance. Hold the contracted position (known as *isometric contraction*) for 10–20 seconds and then release, drawing the foot further into inversion.

## Tips

Perform the action with your wrist locked and move your elbow and trunk to create the force.

## Points to note

There are three peronei muscles (longus, brevis and tertius). Longus and brevis evert the foot and plantarflex while tertius everts and dorsiflexes. Altering the angle of the ankle from neutral to plantarflexion therefore targets the peroneus tertius.

## Exercise 6.32 Anterior tibial acupressure

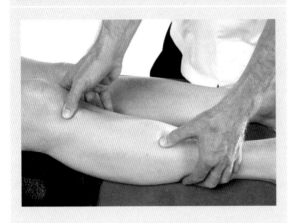

### Purpose

To reduce pain resulting from anterior tibial syndrome (front shin splint) using acupressure.

### Preparation

Begin with your client lying. The stomach meridian is targeted (*see* figure 6.6) stretching from the outer 'eye' of the knee, or the shallow hollow, to the outside of the kneecap tendon (lateral infrapatellar sulcus) to the centre of the ankle joint. Point ST-36 lies three finger widths down from the outer eye and one finger width lateral to the sharp anterior crest of the tibia. This point is often tender to palpation. Three finger widths further down lies ST-37 and at the midpoint of the tibia, equidistant between the knee and ankle, lies ST-38. In the centre of the ankle joint line between the medial and lateral malleolus lies ST-40.

### Action

Locate and compress each point for 2 seconds, repeating the action two or three times along the stomach meridian from knee to ankle.

### Tips

Use deeper pressure over the fleshy points (ST-36/37/38) and less pressure over the bony point (ST-40).

### Points to note

The stomach meridian passes into the foot to travel between the first and second toes and finishes at the lateral side of the base of the second toenail (ST-45). Clients will often feel a dull ache spreading into this area during treatment. The phenomenon is called deqi in Chinese medicine and represents sensory propagation along the channel. This is a feeling which can be quite different between clients. Some may feel a dull ache, others a slight warmth or pleasant tingling sensation. Not all clients feel this, but when they do the treatment result (pain relief, increased circulation, for example) is generally better. The reason for this is that in Traditional Chinese Medicine (TCM) the flow of qi (life force) is essential to health. When the qi flow is interrupted (qi stagnation) tissues are starved of life force and may degenerate. This is a little like watering your garden with a hosepipe; if you step on the hosepipe and cause a blockage the flow of water is disrupted (known as stagnation) and your plants wither and die. The deqi sensation represents the return of the normal flow of qi to support the healing of tissues (i.e. by unblocking the channel).

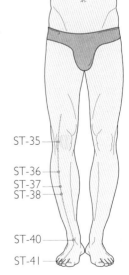

**Figure 6.6** This shows the stomach meridian, used to heal anterior tibial syndrome

**Exercise 6.33** Achilles massage

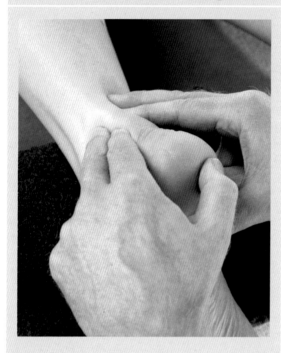

## Purpose
To reduce swelling around the Achilles tendon.

## Preparation
Begin with your client lying face down on a bench with their foot over the bench end. Use the index and middle finger of each hand, curved and pressed together to reinforce each other.

## Action
Use circular friction movements on either side of the Achilles tendon, pressing your fingers together.

## Tips
Work using alternate pressure along the whole length (8–10cm) of the tendon.

## Points to note
Deep pressure into the Achilles can be painful, so keep the pressure light. Also use long effleurage strokes with your fingers (a technique known as *stripping*) to alternate with the circular frictions.

**Exercise 6.34** Achilles, DTF

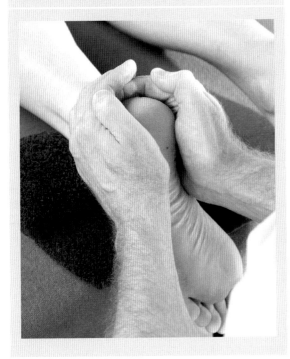

## Purpose

To apply deep transverse friction (DTF) to the under-surface of the Achilles tendon.

## Preparation

Begin with your client lying on their front with their foot pointed (plantarflexed) and supported. Use the thumb of your left hand to press the Achilles to the side. To apply the DTF use the middle finger of your right hand reinforced by your index finger.

## Action

Press your fingers onto the under-surface of the tendon and use a twisting action of your forearm (pronation and supination) to apply the DTF.

## Tips

Apply pressure on the upwards twist (supination) and release pressure on the downward twist (pronation) to allow your fingers to recover.

## Points to note

The inner (medial) aspect of the Achilles is more commonly painful than the outer (lateral).

**Exercise 6.35** DTF to the Achilles tendon insertion

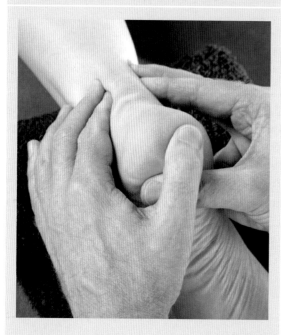

## Purpose

To apply deep transverse friction (DTF) to the Achilles attachment into the heel bone.

## Preparation

Begin with your client lying on their front with their foot bent down (plantarflexed) and top of the foot flat on the bench. Form an 'O' shape with the thumbs and forefingers of both hands.

## Action

Place your thumbs beneath your client's heel and your forefingers (one reinforcing the other) over the top of the heel. Lightly press your forefingers into the base of the Achilles and sway your body weight back to apply force. Move your elbows from side to side to apply the DTF across the Achilles tendon.

## Tips

By swaying your body weight backwards you require very little force to be produced by your fingers; they simply apply the force created by movement of your elbows and body position.

## Points to note

Depending on your client's toe shape they may find their toes pressed into the bench. Where this is the case, place a folded towel between their foot and the bench.

## Exercise 6.36 Lateral ligament, DTF

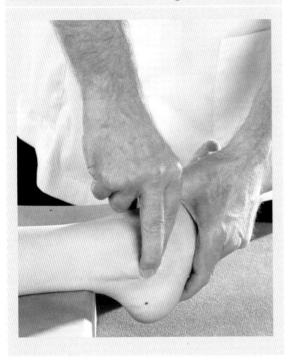

### Purpose

To apply deep transverse friction (DTF) to the lateral ligament of the ankle during the recovery period from ankle sprain.

### Preparation

Begin with your client sitting with their foot close to the bench end. With your left hand, draw their foot downwards and inwards (plantarflexion and inversion). Your massage contact is your index finger supported by your middle finger.

### Action

Apply the DTF by locking your wrist and fingers and moving your elbow. The action is small (1–2cm) and in an almost horizontal direction.

### Tips

Apply force as you draw your fingers downwards, but release the force slightly on the upward stroke to recover.

### Points to note

The front portion (anterior band) of the ligament is more commonly affected, and this angles downwards at 45 degrees from the outer ankle bone (lateral malleolus). Your action should be perpendicular to this line.

**Exercise 6.37** Ankle medial collateral ligament, DTF

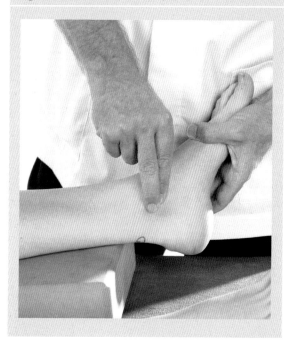

## Purpose

To broaden the fibres of the lateral ankle ligament using deep transverse friction (DTF).

## Preparation

Begin with your client lying with their shin placed over the bench end or on a block. Use one hand to draw the ankle down (plantarflexion) and inwards (inversion). The anterior band of the ligament is located between the anterior border of the ankle bone (lateral malleolus) and the ankle mortise (talus), and is approximately the width of the index finger.

## Action

Apply the DTF at an angle of 45 degrees just in front and below the ankle bone. Apply sufficient pressure so that your fingers do not slide over the skin, and continue the massage for 3–5 minutes.

## Tips

Apply more force on the downward stroke of the massage, releasing slightly and resting your fingers on the upward stroke.

## Points to note

The lateral ligament of the ankle has three bands. The anterior band (anterior talofibular ligament) travels forwards and is almost horizontal in its orientation. This is the most commonly injured section of the ligament and the one targeted using this technique.

## Exercise 6.38 Plantarfascia release

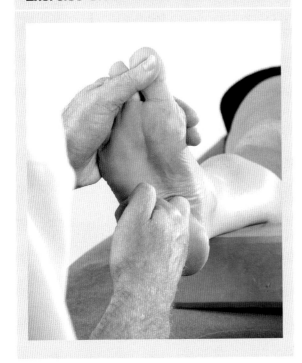

### Purpose

To release tension and pain in the sole of the foot using fascial release (FR).

### Preparation

Begin with your client lying on their back with their heel over the bench end, calf resting on a folded towel. Use the knuckle of your index finger reinforce it with your thumb to provide your massage contact.

### Action

Apply a slow but continuous pressure with your knuckle along the length of the plantarfascia from the heel bone (calcaneus) to the base of the big toe.

### Tips

The pressure is increased if you tighten the plantarfascia by pulling the foot downwards (plantarflexion) and bending the toe up (first ray extension).

### Points to note

As an active soft tissue release (STR), press your knuckle into the plantarfascia and keep it still as your client bends and straightens their big toe.

### Exercise 6.39 Intermetatarsal, DTM

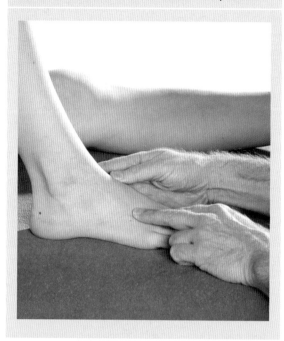

### Purpose

To release tension within the interosseous muscles between the toes using deep tissue massage (DTM).

### Preparation

Begin with your client lying with their knees bent and foot flat. Use the pad of one finger supported by the other as your massage contact.

### Action

Use an even pressure into the gap between the toes. Apply straight compression and then circular frictional massage to mobilise the tissues locally.

### Tips

Where the toes have been pressed tightly together by ill fitting footwear, use one hand to draw the toes apart and apply massage with the other hand.

### Points to note

The digital nerves run between the toe bones (metatarsals). Pressure onto the nerves through clinical massage can cause tingling into the toes which stops when massage has finished.

# TRUNK TECHNIQUES

7

## ANATOMY REFRESHER

The trunk consists of the spine and ribcage. The spine itself is divided into cervical (neck) thoracic (mid) and lumbar (lower) regions, with the sacrum and coccyx forming the rudiments of your tail. The spinal column is made up of 33 individual bones (vertebrae). Each vertebra is numbered to show its position. Cervical vertebra numbers begin with 'C', thoracic 'T', lumbar 'L' and sacral 'S'. So the second cervical vertebra, for example, counting down from the head is C2, and the fourth C4. The last lumbar vertebra is L5 (rather than L1) because the numbering system begins at the head each time (*see* figure 7.2).

## BONE STRUCTURES OF THE TRUNK

The cervical region is subdivided into two parts. The upper portion directly below your head is called the *sub-occipital region* (the occiput being the lower portion of the back of your skull). The C1 and C2 bones make up this region and these two bones are intimately related with skull movements, especially nodding actions. The lower portion of the neck is called the *lower cervical region* and takes in the bones C3 through to C7. This region is more involved with twisting (rotation) and side bending (lateral flexion) actions.

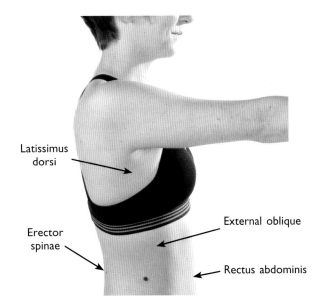

Latissimus dorsi

Erector spinae

External oblique

Rectus abdominis

**Figure 7.1** The anatomy of the trunk

---

### Keypoint

Vertebrae are numbered from the head down, with C1 just below the head and C7 between the shoulders.

In the chest region the bones are called *thoracic* vertebrae and these bones connect to the ribs via small joints (*see* below). In the lower spine the spinal bones are called *lumbar* vertebrae. These are large and strong bones covered with powerful muscles. They do not attach to the ribs but their movements are intimately linked to those of the pelvis. The upper portion of the lumbar spine, L1 and L2, move with the thoracic spine, especially during shoulder blade and ribcage movements. The lower lumbar vertebrae, L3, 4 and 5, move closely with the pelvis so that this combined region is often referred to as the *lumbo-pelvis*.

Below the lumbar vertebrae are the remnants of our tail. The *sacrum* is a triangular shaped bone which attaches at the sides to the pelvis, while the *coccyx* forms a thin pointed tip to the end of the spine (*see* figure 7.2). Both of these regions are important because they can be prone to injury during pregnancy and childbirth. The joint between the sacrum and the pelvis (sacroiliac joint, *see* figure 7.2) is filled with fibrous material and normally gives little movement. During childbirth, however, the fibrous material softens and the joint moves to allow the pelvis to expand, thereby facilitating childbirth. The coccyx again becomes more mobile in this period and can become problematic. In addition, in the lean individual the coccyx is easily damaged by sitting or falling backwards directly onto a hard floor.

## Keypoint

The sacroiliac joint joins the sacrum to the pelvis. It is often painful during pregnancy and following childbirth.

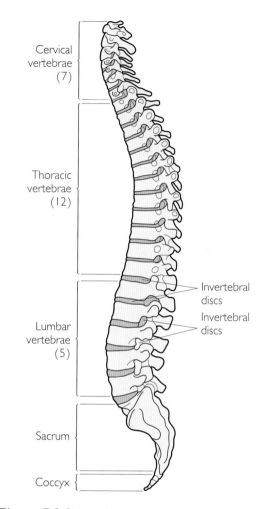

**Figure 7.2** Below the lumbar vertebrae: the coccyx, the sacrum and the sacroiliac joint

## Spinal curves

Although the spinal vertebrae stand one on top of each other, the column they make is not straight. Rather the spine forms an 'S' curve. There are two inward curves in the lower back and neck, while the thoracic spine curves gently outwards. The inward curves are called the lumbar lordosis and cervical lordosis, while the outward curve is the thoracic kyphosis.

When a client lies down on a treatment bench it is often necessary to support the curves with a rolled towel or pad to make them feel more comfortable. In addition, the curves may increase or reduce through injury, stiffness or muscle spasm. Massage which relaxes spasm may cause the spinal curves to change.

## The spinal segment

Each pair of spinal bones together forms a single unit called a *spinal segment* (*see* figure 7.3). The two bones are separated by a spongy disc attached to the flat part of the bone. At the back of the vertebra the bone is extended to form two small joints called *facets*. From above it can be seen that the back of the spinal bone forms a hollow arch through which runs the spinal cord, which carries messages from the brain to the legs and arms (*see* figure 7.4).

Gym users tend to talk about whole spine movements when bending and straightening, often without realising that segments of the spine can move relative to each other. Instructors look

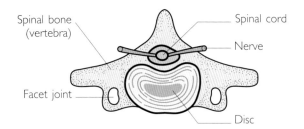

**Figure 7.4** The spinal cord runs through the spinal bone

at specific segments of motion; for example, during an overhead shoulder exercise the thoracic spine may be flattening while the lumbar spine curves excessively. Therapists look in even closer detail at the individual spinal segments. They are interested in the motion between L5/L4 relative to that of L4/L3, for example, because the motion of an individual spinal segment can provide useful information. Stiffness in one segment following injury may cause a neighbouring segment to move excessively (known as *compensatory hypermobility*), causing pain. The answer to this is to make the stiff segment move more so that the lax segment can move less. A physiotherapist will often use joint manipulation to release a stiff spinal segment and then exercise therapy to re-educate the muscles supporting the lax segment.

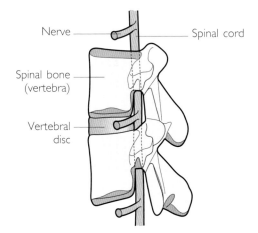

**Figure 7.3** Each pair of spinal bones together forms a single unit called a spinal segment

### Keypoint

Look closer at spinal movements. Notice movement of (a) the whole spine, (b) regions of the spine relative to each other and (c) individual spinal segments. These can give you valuable information about the client's condition.

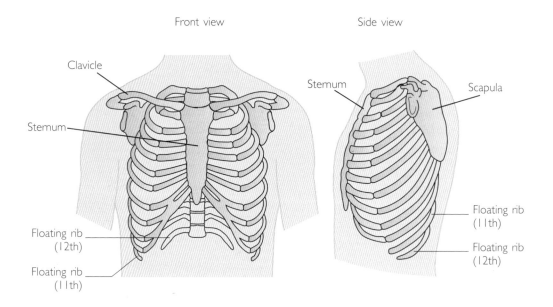

Front view     Side view

Clavicle

Sternum

Sternum

Scapula

Floating rib
(12th)

Floating rib
(11th)

Floating rib
(11th)

Floating rib
(12th)

**Figure 7.5** The lower two ribs are not attached to the sternum at the front and are known as 'floating ribs'

## Ribcage

The ribcage is formed of 12 sets of ribs on each side of the body. These connect to the thoracic spine at the back and the breast bone (sternum) at the front. Anything to do with the ribs is called costo in medical terms, so the joint with the sternum is the *sternocostal* (SC) joint, that with the vertebra is the *costovertebral* (CV) joint and that with the side bone (known as the transverse process) of the vertebra is the *costotransverse* (CT) joint. The lower two ribs (11 and 12) are not attached to the sternum at the front, but float free and are therefore called floating ribs (*see* figure 7.5).

When looking at someone's back, the spinous processes are in the middle, forming a straight column of bumps. The CV joint is about two finger breaths to the side, lying in the furrow of the back. The CT joint is about three finger breadths to the side, covered by the large erector spinae muscles. The rib curves at the rib angle to form the drum of the chest (*see* figure 7.6).

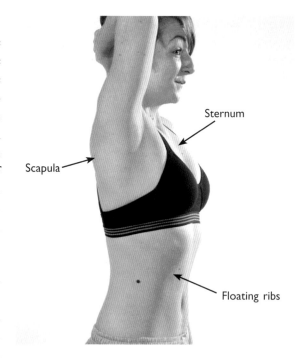

Sternum

Scapula

Floating ribs

**Figure 7.6** The rib curves at the rib angle to form the drum of the chest

114

# MUSCLE STRUCTURES OF THE TRUNK

The back muscles consist of two groups, those which run the whole length of your spine (multisegmental) and those running just between two neighbouring vertebrae (unisegmental).

## Multisegmental muscles of the trunk

The *erector spinae muscles* form the first group and these run from the rim of your pelvis along the side of your spine. They consist of two portions; firstly long muscles close to the spine (known as longissimus) and secondly muscles further away from the spine which fan out to the ribs (iliocostalis). A further muscle (quadratus lumborum) attaches from the rim of your pelvis to your lower ribs. These are powerful muscles lying relatively close to the body surface, and they respond well to massage techniques. They often develop trigger points and can be a common source of pain from back conditions.

## Unisegmental muscles of the trunk

The second muscle group consists of small local muscles attaching between the spinous processes (interspinalis), transverse processes (intertransversus) and at the side of the spine in small blocks (multifidus). Importantly these muscles are more deeply placed and harder to work on during clinical massage therapy.

At the front of the trunk are the abdominal muscles, consisting of the central strip of block-like muscles (rectus abdominis) and the oblique abdominal surrounding the trunk (internal and external obliques). Beneath these you have a sheet of muscle (transversus) which encircles the trunk and attaches to your back fascia. For further details of trunk muscle structure and function see *The Complete Guide to Abdominal Training* (Norris 2009).

## Exercise 7.1 Back fascial stretch

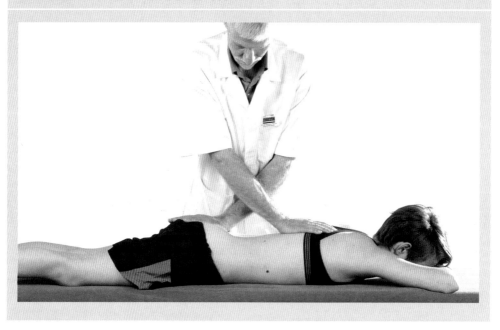

### Purpose
To lengthen the back (thoracolumbar) fascia.

### Preparation
Begin with your client lying on their front (you will not need massage cream). Cross your arms and place your hands flat on your client's back, your lower (known as *caudal*) hand with fingers pointing to your client's feet and your upper (*cephalic*) hand with fingers pointing to their head.

### Action
Keeping your elbows locked, lean your body weight forwards, which will cause your arms to press apart. Do not allow your hands to slip over the skin surface as this can cause painful friction

### Tips
To reduce the pressure of this stretch, do not lean as far forwards – slightly flex your elbows instead. Allow the stretch to build up, easing into the movement and prolonging the stretch for 5–10 seconds to allow tissue change.

### Points to note
If your client's lumbar curve (lordosis) is deep, place a folded towel beneath their abdomen.

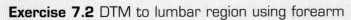

## Exercise 7.2 DTM to lumbar region using forearm

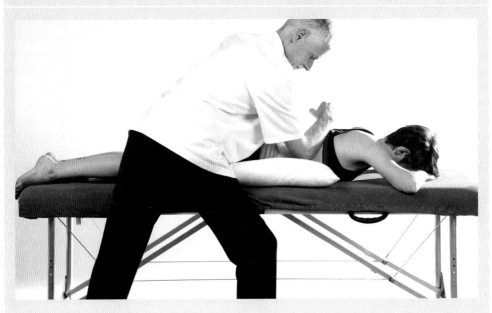

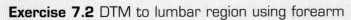

### Purpose

To give deep tissue massage (DTM) to the superficial back muscles.

### Preparation

Begin with your client lying on their front. Use the side of your forearm as your massage contact, and use massage cream or gel rather than oil. Oil is too thin and slippy and will not allow you to press deeply into the tissues. The depth of your force (a vertical motion) will simply slide away (in a horizontal motion).

### Action

Place the side of your forearm onto your client and lean your body forwards to produce the required amount of pressure. Press your forearm sideways (longitudinally), allowing it to slowly move across the skin surface.

### Tips

Raise or lower your elbow to keep your forearm in contact with your client's skin surface as you move.

### Points to note

Reduce pressure over the rib area and increase pressure over the thick erector spinae muscles, as they attach to the sacrum and pelvis because treatment of the muscle rather than the rib is the aim of this technique.

## Exercise 7.3 Acupressure to lumbar spine

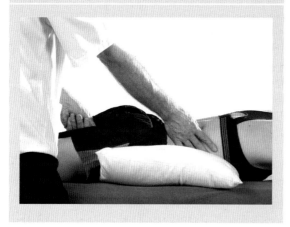

## Purpose

To reduce pain and spasm in the lumbar region using acupressure.

## Preparation

Begin with your client lying on their front, with a folded towel or thin pillow beneath their abdomen.

## Action

The acupuncture channel (meridian) most commonly used for low back pain is the bladder (BL) channel. This has two branches on either side of the spine – the inner bladder channel lies two finger widths from the centre of the spinous processes, the outer channel one hand width from the centre, approximately level with the inner edge of the shoulder blade (otherwise known as the medial border of scapula). The bladder channel travels down the back of the thigh and the two channels join at the back of the knee at the point BL-40 lying on the knee joint line at the midpoint between the inner and outer hamstring tendons (semitendinosus and biceps femoris). The channel travels between the bellies of the large calf muscle (gastrocnemius) and to the outside of the ankle. BL-57 lies at the midpoint between the ankle and knee, BL-60 between the outer ankle bone (lateral malleolus) and the Achilles tendon (*see* figure 7.7).

Use a single knuckle (reinforced) to apply pressure to the acupuncture points of the inner bladder line, pressing at the highest point of the erector spinae muscles (longissimus portion). Target painful points, but also use the classical acupuncture point BL-23 on either side of the body. This point lies level with the second lumbar vertebra (L2). Also apply pressure to BL-40, BL-57 and BL-60 to increase energy (qi) flow along the acupuncture channel.

## Tips

You may also treat your client in sitting position with their arms supported at chest height on the cushions placed on the bench (forward lean sitting), to target the back points.

## Points to note

As you apply pressure do so gradually, avoiding any sudden lunging action.

**Figure 7.7** The meridian most commonly used for low back pain is the bladder (BL) channel

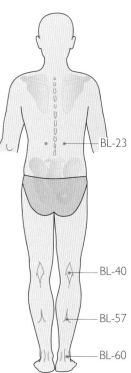

## Exercise 7.4 Erector spinae TrPs

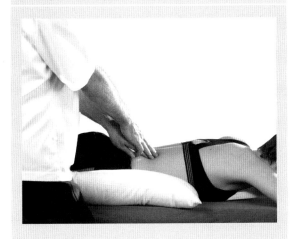

### Purpose
To reduce pain and spasm within the erector spinae muscles.

### Preparation
Begin with your client lying on their front, with a folded towel or thin pillow beneath their abdomen.

### Action
Begin using general massage strokes to relax the local area and to assess tissue tension. Identify a trigger point (TrP) as a tight band or nodule within the erector spinae muscles. Press into the nodule using a gradually increasing (crescendo) pressure. Hold the pressure for 30–120 seconds and then release slowly.

### Tips
As the pressure is deep and sustained, use your knuckle or a massage tool to reduce stress on your fingers.

### Points to note
It is normal for local pain to increase at the start of this procedure. Pain should stabilise and gradually subside as point pressure is maintained.

### Exercise 7.5 Quadratus lumborum TrPs

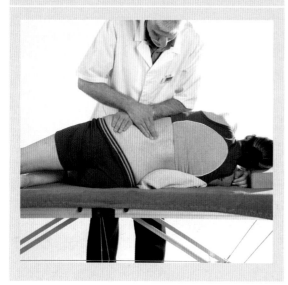

## Purpose

To release local pain and spasm within the quadratus lumborum (QL) muscles.

## Preparation

Begin with your client lying on the unaffected side. Place a rolled towel or cushion beneath their trunk to side flex them towards you. This body position will place the QL on stretch, as side flexion increases the distance between the ribs and pelvis, the two areas to which the muscle attaches.

## Action

Begin using local massage to relax the region and assess tissue tension. Identify the QL running between the rim of the pelvis (iliac crest) to the lower ribs. Massage into the area to identify a TrP as a tight band or nodule lying within the muscle. Press into the nodule using an increasing pressure. Hold the pressure for 30–120 seconds and then release slowly.

## Tips

As the pressure is deep and sustained, use your knuckle, fingers pressed together, or a massage tool to reduce stress on your fingers.

## Points to note

Allowing the upper leg to cross over the lower will dip the pelvis slightly and increase the side flexed position.

## Exercise **7.6** Quadratus lumborum STR with hip hitch

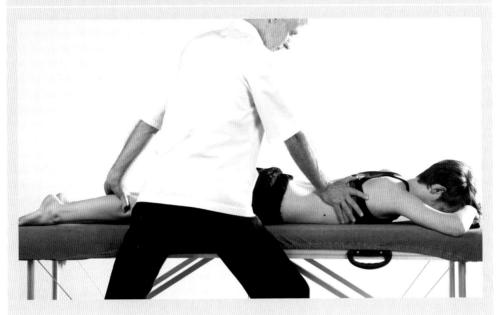

### Purpose
To release the quadratus lumborum (QL) muscle using active soft tissue release (STR).

### Preparation
Begin with your client lying on their front with their feet over the bench end.

### Action
Apply pressure using the knuckles of one hand reinforced by the other. Press into the tight QL area and instruct your client to lengthen and then shorten the leg on the painful side, keeping the leg straight.

### Tips
In this action your hand should stay still, the movement being produced by your client's hip hitching action.

### Points to note
The hip hitch action contracts and then relaxes the QL to induce muscle relaxation (known as post-isometric relaxation).

**Exercise 7.7** Multifidus TrPs

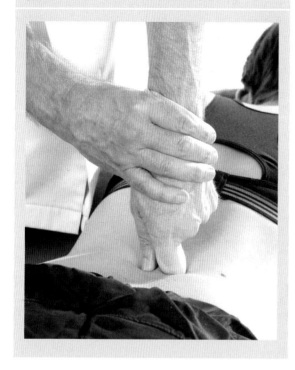

### Purpose
To release pain and tension close to the spine.

### Preparation
Begin with your client lying on their front with a cushion beneath their abdomen to flatten their spine. Your massage contact should be your reinforced fingertips or a 'V' shape formed by the knuckle of your index finger and the tip of your thumb.

### Action
Locate the multifidus muscle at the side of your client's spinous processes. Press into the tight area using a gradually increasing pressure. Hold the pressure for 30–120 seconds and then slowly release.

### Tips
This technique may also be performed with your client kneeling, with their arms forwards.

### Points to note
The multifidus is a small block-like muscle lying within the channel between the spinous processes and the bulky erector spinae muscles, known as the *paraspinal gutter*.

## Exercise 7.8 DTM to erector spinae in sitting flexion

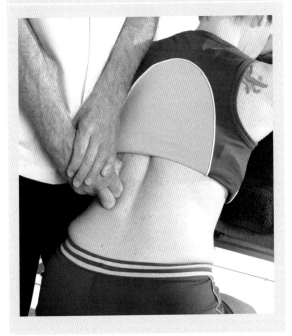

### Purpose

To release tension within the erector spinae muscles using point pressure deep tissue massage (DTM) in sitting.

### Preparation

Begin with your client sitting on a stool or side on to a chair. Support their upper body on a stack of cushions on a table top or bench. This should be high enough to allow them to fold their arms and rest their forehead on the backs of their hands. Stand behind your client and use your knuckles as a massage contact.

### Action

Contact the erector spinae muscles with two or more knuckles initially to broaden your contact area. Power for the action comes from a lunge stance position, taking your body weight from your back foot to your front.

### Tips

Tuck your elbow into your side to stabilise your arm as you work.

### Points to note

You will need to sink low through your knees to keep your own back straight as you work on your client's lower (lumbar) spine. Straighten up as you work higher up their spine into the thoracic region.

**Exercise 7.9** Spinal rotation, MET in sitting

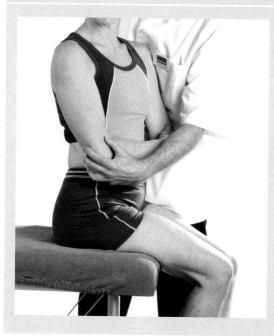

## Purpose

To release spinal muscle spasm and regain rotation symmetry using muscle energy technique (MET).

## Preparation

Begin with your client sitting on the end of the treatment bench or on a low stool (gym bench). Ask them to fold their arms, lightly gripping their elbows.

## Action

Ask your client to turn their trunk to the right as far as spasm/pain allows. Get them to move only to the point where pain/stiffness begins (engages). Grasp their shoulders and try to press them further into range while they resist the action (known as *isometric muscle contraction*). Maintain the muscle tension for 10–20 seconds and then release. Gently move them further into their range and stop once more when pain/stiffness begins. Repeat the action to the other direction.

## Tips

As you apply pressure make sure the direction is horizontal to cause pure rotation, not partially downwards, which would cause rotation and flexion.

## Points to note

It is common for asymmetry to occur with rotation in one direction being greater than the other. Symmetry (equal range to both sides) may take several sessions to develop, because movement range may be limited by soft tissue resistance other than muscle spasm.

## Exercise 7.10 Spinal side flexion, MET in side lying

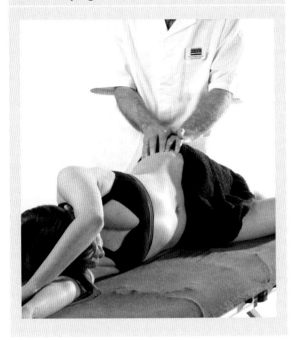

### Purpose

To release spinal muscle spasm and regain side flexion symmetry using muscle energy technique (MET).

### Preparation

Begin with your client lying on their unaffected side. Their shins should be level with the end of the bench, feet dropped over the end. Flex the bottom leg and allow the top leg to lower into adduction. Reach their top arm overhead to lengthen the latissimus dorsi and thoracolumbar fascia (TLF). Stand at the bench end with your legs astride your client's leg and grip the rim of their pelvis in your interlinked hands.

### Action

Ask your client to simultaneously lift their leg into abduction to the horizontal and hitch their hip using the instruction 'shorten your top leg'. Follow the pelvic movement with your hands, applying minimal resistance. Hold the contracted position for 10–15 seconds and then release. As their leg lowers back into adduction, draw their pelvis towards you, side flexing their spine.

### Tips

Resistance for the action is largely provided by your client lifting their leg into abduction. The minimal resistance to their pelvis provides them with feedback (known as tactile feedback) for the hip hitch action.

### Points to note

Your aim is to increase the distance between your client's lower ribs and their pelvis on the targeted side.

**Exercise 7.11** Intercostal muscle, STR

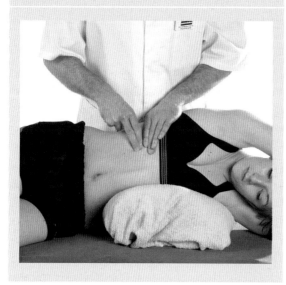

## Purpose

To reduce muscle pain between the ribs using soft tissue release (STR).

## Preparation

Begin with your client lying on their side over a pillow to open their ribs. Use a single reinforced finger as your massage contact.

## Action

Massage between the ribs, initially using a circling technique. Next, have your client breathe in deeply to expand their ribcage while you press down with the side of your hand onto one rib. Repeat this action for several ribs within a tight area.

## Tips

The action is a gentle pressure, aiming to hold the lower rib down as your client lifts the upper rib during deep inspiration.

## Points to note

Perform a maximum of three movements with your client breathing deeply, and then allow them to breathe normally for 20–30 seconds. Breathing in deeply too many times can cause your client to hyperventilate and go light headed.

**Exercise 7.12** Sub-occipital, STR

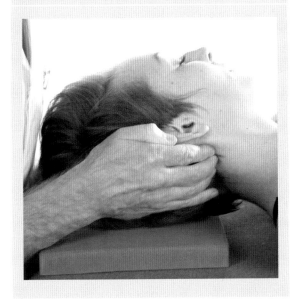

## Purpose
To release tension in the soft tissues attaching to the base of the skull using soft tissue release (STR).

## Preparation
Begin with your client lying on their back with their head on a folded towel. You should sit at the head end of the bench and place your forearms beneath their head.

## Action
Use your fingertips as your massage contact and focus on two alternating techniques. Swivel (pronate and supinate) your forearms to impose a deep transverse friction (DTF) to the sub-occipital muscles, and bend (flex) your fingers to impart STR.

## Tips
The action should be slow and flowing to aid muscle relaxation.

## Points to note
The weight of your client's head pressing down onto your fingers negates the need for you to use force. Do not press upwards into their suboccipital tissues, but allow their head weight to press down onto your fingers.

**Exercise 7.13** Cervical traction, STR

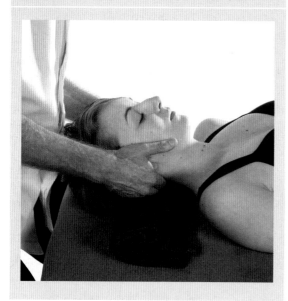

### Purpose
To lengthen and release the cervical soft tissues using soft tissue release (STR).

### Preparation
Begin with your client lying face up on a bench. Their head should be straight (aligned). If your client has a head forward (protracted) posture, their head may fall back onto the bench, so place a small block or folded towel beneath it.

### Action
Sitting behind your client, grip their head with your fingers beneath the back of their skull (occiput) and thumbs behind their ears (known as the *mastoid process*). Slowly draw their head towards you, encouraging their neck to become longer, almost imperceptibly.

### Tips
Use only 1–2lb of force, the same amount as you would choose to gently stretch a sore muscle.

### Points to note
Make sure your pulling pressure (traction) is applied evenly. There is a tendency to pull harder on the back of the skull and tip the head backwards.

**Exercise 7.14** Cervical rotation, MET

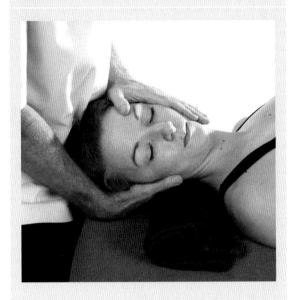

## Purpose
To regain symmetry of rotation motion range using muscle energy technique (MET).

## Preparation
Begin with your client lying face up on a bench. Their head should be aligned. If your client has a head forward posture, place a small block or folded towel beneath their head.

## Action
Lightly grip your client's head with your fingers beneath their skull and your thumbs to the sides. Firstly, assess their rotation range by supporting their head as they turn it to the right and left. Next, ask them to turn their head to their stiffer side and when you get to their maximum range, hold their head and ask them to turn back against your resistance. Hold this gentle tension (isometric contraction) for 10–20 seconds and then release. Reassess their motion range.

## Tips
Your client leads this action, while you merely support the weight of their head.

## Points to note
This action uses a contract-relax stretching method to release tension in your client's neck muscles. Your aim is only to guide their movement – never force the turning (rotation) movement of your client's head as it can cause severe injury.

### Exercise 7.15 Sub-occipital MET using head retraction

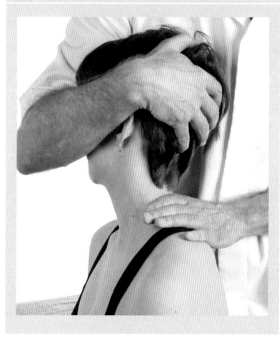

## Purpose

To release tension in the sub-occipital region and facilitate head retraction using muscle energy technique (MET).

## Preparation

Begin with your client sitting on a low stool or treatment bench. Stand to the right side of them and wrap your right arm around their head, resting their forehead against your ribcage and right upper arm. Grip the back of their head in your curved hand, and use the side of the forefinger of your left hand against their cervical spine to stabilise this region.

## Action

Press your arm forwards to encourage backward sliding (retraction) of your client's head on their non-moving neck. Press in a horizontal direction only, avoiding flexion or extension. Stop at the point where you feel tissue resistance or your client experiences pain. Ask them to tighten their muscles to resist your pressure (known as *isometric contraction*). Hold this tension for 10–20 seconds and then repeat.

## Tips

Place a paper towel between your client's face and your arm/chest for hygiene purposes.

## Points to note

The sub-occipital portion of the cervical spine is the upper part (C1–C3). To stabilise the lower portion of the neck, press the forefinger of your left hand below this level. In this way the sub-occipital region is able to move on a firmer base.

## Exercise 7.16 Jaw trigger point and acupressure release

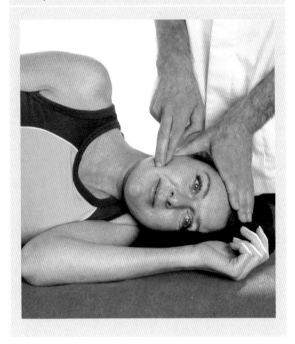

masseter (one of the muscles of mastication). ST-8 lies on a vertical line joining ST-6 and ST-7, just back from the hairline at the thickest part of the temporalis muscle.

### Action
Once the acupuncture points have been located, palpate around the local area for a thickened and painful area which represents the trigger point (TrP). Press the point for 10–30 seconds until pain and local tissue tension subsides.

### Tips
The muscles are quite thin, so very little pressure is required for effective treatment.

### Points to note
It is common for pain to refer into your client's jaw as you press these points. Pain should ease gradually. If it does not, release pressure and rest for 1 minute before repeating.

### Purpose
To release tension in the jaw muscles following teeth grinding or temporomandibular joint (TMJ) pain using acupressure release.

### Preparation
Begin with your client lying on their painless side. Place one or two folded towels between the side of their head and the bench to align their neck and prevent side bending. The stomach meridian is targeted, with points ST-7, ST-6 and ST-8 being used (*see* figure 7.8). ST-7 lies just in front of the jaw joint (mandibular condyle) and is also a trigger point for the lateral pterygoid muscle. ST-6 lies one finger width diagonally forwards from the jaw angle and is a trigger point for the

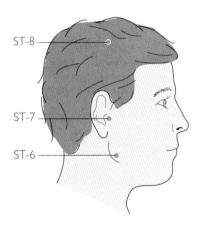

**Figure 7.8** The acupressure points used to treat jaw pain

## Exercise **7.17** Facial acupressure techniques

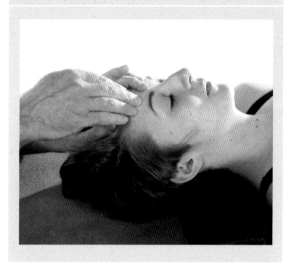

### Purpose
To release tension within the facial muscles and stimulate local blood flow.

### Preparation
Begin with your client lying flat, with a folded towel beneath their head to align the neck. Stand behind, at the head end of the bench, and target the following acupressure points GB-14, ST-3, SI-18 on both sides of the body (bilateral) and yintang and CV-24 unilaterally (*see* figure 7.9). GB-14 lies one finger width above the centre of the eyebrow, ST-3 in line with the centre of the eye at the side of the nose, SI-18 over the cheek bone (zygoma), in line with the outer edge of the eye. The point yintang is directly between the eyebrows and CV-24 in the centre of the groove below the lower lip.

### Action
Press each point and hold the pressure for 20–30 seconds. Treat each bilateral and unilateral point in sequence from the top of the face to the bottom and repeat the sequence three times.

### Tips
Where a person holds tension in their face the points may be painful to pressure, but the pain should ease as the point is treated.

### Points to note
The feeling from the acupuncture point may spread. This sensation is called deqi in acupuncture, and represents sensory propagation along the acupuncture channel.

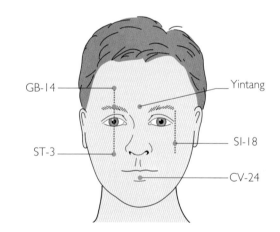

**Figure 7.9** The acupressure points on the face

**Exercise 7.18** Rhomboid TrP release

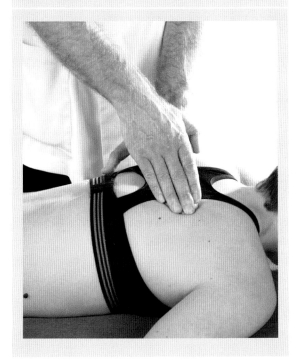

### Purpose

To reduce pain and discomfort between the shoulder blades using trigger point (TrP) release.

### Preparation

Begin with your client lying on their front, with the painful arm over the bench side.

### Action

Locate the rhomboid muscles between the spine and inner aspect (medial border) of the shoulder blade (scapula). Use one or two fingers supported by your thumb as a massage contact. Gently press into the tender area, allowing the tight tissues to release gradually over 10–20 seconds.

### Tips

The rhomboids are thin muscles so make sure that you pressure them with the flat surface of your finger (shaft of the phalanx) rather than your knuckle (interphalangeal joint) as this will be less painful for the client.

### Points to note

Placing your client's arm over the bench side draws the shoulder blade of the painful side away from their spine (abduction), stretching the rhomboid muscles.

**Exercise 7.19** Upper trapezius, DTM in sitting

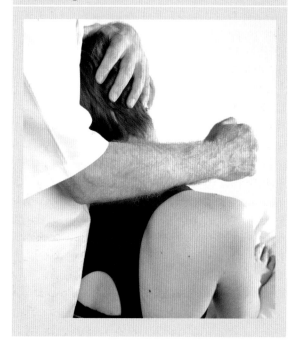

## Purpose

To release tension in the upper fibres of the trapezius muscle using deep tissue massage (DTM).

## Preparation

Begin with your client sitting upright in a chair with their arm supported on a cushion. Stand at their painful side and slightly behind them. Use your forearm as your massage contact.

## Action

To massage your client's right shoulder, stabilise with your left hand and massage using your right forearm. Press your forearm across and then upward in a half 'U' shape, following the contour of the muscle.

## Tips

Reduce pressure as you move from the shoulder (horizontal motion) to the neck (vertical motion).

## Points to note

It is normal for your client's head to move away from you slightly as you apply pressure. However, if they markedly side flex their neck, your pressure is too great.

**Exercise 7.20** Levator scapulae, STR

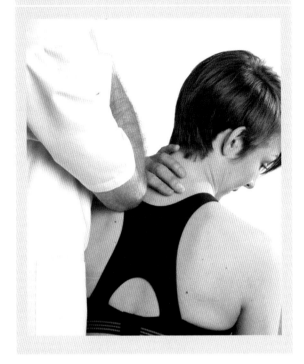

### Purpose
To target the levator scapulae muscle running from the inner top of the shoulder blade (scapular superior angle) to the neck using soft tissue release (STR).

### Preparation
Begin with your client sitting upright in a chair with their arm supported on a cushion. Stand at their painful side and slightly behind them. Use your elbow as your massage contact.

### Action
Begin by applying deep tissue massage(DTM) to the levator just above the point of the shoulder. Work in slowly to encourage the muscle to release (reduce tone). Next, apply a STR lock by fixing the muscle with your elbow and encouraging your client to lengthen the muscle by looking down and away from your elbow (cervical flexion, lateral rotation and side flexion away from the pain).

### Tips
Point pressure onto the muscle can be quite painful as it is thin and lies directly on the ribcage. Begin with mild pressure, only increasing in intensity as your client's tissues relax.

### Points to note
The position of your elbow when applying the lock will also fix the shoulder blade in a downwards direction (depression).

**Exercise 7.21** Pectoral release lying

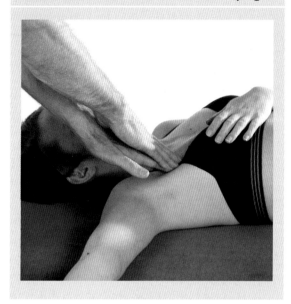

## Purpose

To release tension in the powerful pectoral muscles which tighten in a round shouldered (kyphotic) posture.

## Preparation

Begin with your client lying on their back close to the edge of the bench while you stand to the other side of the bench. Move their arm to the side (abduction) to begin placing the muscle on stretch. Use your fist or two fingers reinforced by your thumb.

## Action

Begin using direct pressure massage into the pectorals from the breastbone (sternum) to the upper arm (humerus).

## Tips

You may use a soft tissue release (STR) in this position by holding your client's arm upwards (adducted position, fixing your hand on their pectoral muscle and then moving their arm outwards (abduction).

## Points to note

A female client should place her opposite hand over her breast on the painful side to protect modesty.

**Exercise 7.22** Erector spinae, active STR in sitting

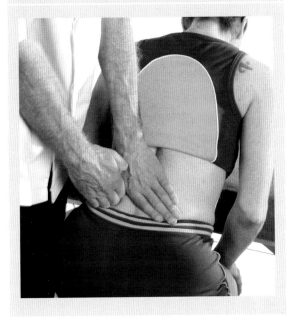

## Purpose

To target the erector spinae muscles using an active soft tissue release (STR).

## Preparation

Begin with your client sitting on a stool, or side on to a chair. Your massage contact is the knuckles of your index and middle fingers of each hand pressed together to form a long 'V' shape. The centre of the 'V' is placed over your client spinous processes, with the shaft of the middle fingers (middle phalanx) contacting the erector spinae muscles (longissimus).

## Action

Keep your arms straight and press your knuckles into the muscles. Hold this position and ask your client to bend (flex) their spine, initiating the movement from their head and shoulders.

## Tips

Use a lunge stance (*see* page 32), so you can transfer your body weight from your back to your front foot as you follow the movement of your client's spine.

## Points to note

Make sure your client does not lean forwards as they bend their spine. The action is to draw their nose to their tummy button (umbilicus) rather than towards the floor.

**Exercise 7.23** Sitting side flexion, STR

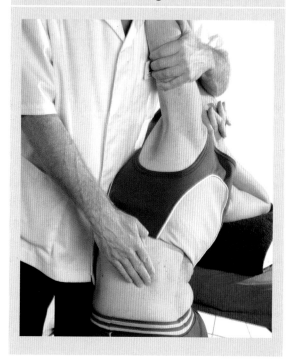

## Purpose

To release the side flexor muscle and increase motion range using soft tissue release (STR).

## Preparation

Begin with your client sitting on a stool close to the side of a bench or table, with their hands behind their head.

## Action

Ask your client to side-bend away from their painful side, and adjust the bench so that they can rest their near arm onto the bench. Support their upper arm, and apply massage and fascial stretch to the side of their trunk.

## Tips

If your client is unable to comfortably place their hands behind their head they may put the backs of their hands on their forehead.

## Points to note

This action is a combination of downward pressure to stretch the fascia, and upwards pressure on the arm to lengthen the tissue as it releases.

## Summary of key terms

- **Caudal** Closer to the tail
- **Cephalic** Closer to the head

# CHEST AND ABDOMEN TECHNIQUES

8

We have looked at the ribcage from the back, where the ribs attach to the thoracic vertebrae (*see* page 114), and now we will look from the front to observe conditions affecting the chest and abdomen.

For the abdomen, clinical massage can be used to target two groups of structures. The first group is *muscular* and consists of the abdominal muscles which we will look at here, the second group is *visceral* (organs). These are targeted both by traditional massage techniques for constipation, and by specialist visceral mobilisation, which is outside the remit of this book. For details of visceral manipulation see J. P. Barral's book *Visceral Manipulation* (Eastland Press 2008) or visit www.barralinstitute.co.uk.

## RIBCAGE

We have seen in chapter 7 that the ribcage is formed by 12 sets of ribs on each side of the body. These connect to the thoracic spine at the back and the breast bone (sternum) at the front, forming the sternocostal (SC) joints. The lower two ribs (11 and 12) are not attached to the sternum at the front, but float free and constitute the floating ribs. Between the ribs there are three muscles called the *intercostals* (external, internal,

innermost) which open and close the rib spaces as you breath. Lying in a small groove beneath the rib (*intercostal groove*) are the intercostal nerve, artery and vein. Pain can travel along the ribs via the intercostal nerve, while damage to the ribs can cause local bruising when blood vessels rupture.

## ABDOMINAL MUSCLES

The abdominals consist of both superficial (surface) and deep muscles.

Superficially the central strip of the abdomen is a block-like muscle, known as the *rectus abdominis*. This muscle runs from the lower ribs to the pubic region, forming a narrow strap which tapers down from about 15cm wide at the top to 8cm at the bottom. The muscle has three fibrous bands across it (*tendonous intersections*) at the level of the tummy button, and above and below this point. The rectus muscle on each side of the body is contained within a sheath (*rectus sheath*), the two sheaths merging in the centre line of the body via a strong fibrous band called the *linea alba*. During pregnancy the muscle must stretch to accommodate the developing baby, but as the development is so fast the muscle cannot keep up and so the linea alba splits to form a gap (*diastasis recti*) in the last third of pregnancy (third trimester). The condition is more common during a woman's second or third pregnancy as the muscles have already stretched by that point. The diastasis should resolve naturally in the months following childbirth, but in some cases women can be left with a gap between the two muscles or a line of flattened scar tissue. Surgery (usually a tummy tuck) may be required in extreme cases, where the linea is folded and then stitched together.

### Keypoint

In late pregnancy the central band between the two rectus muscles will broaden creating a *diastasis recti*. This can sometimes remain separated after childbirth.

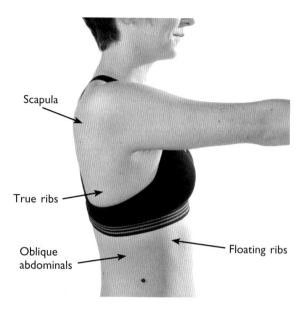

**Figure 8.1** Chest and abdomen anatomy

Winding across the abdomen are the oblique abdominal muscles (*internal and external obliques*). The internal oblique travels from the pubic region (pelvic bone and *inguinal ligament*) up and across to the lower ribs and into the rectus sheath. The external oblique is more superficial, but has a similar position lying at an angle to the internal oblique. It travels from the lower ribs to the rectus and then to the pubic area. The fibres in the centre of the external oblique lie diagonally, but those right on the edge lie vertically.

Underneath the oblique abdominals lies the *transversus abdominis* muscle. This attaches from the pelvic bones and tissue covering the spinal muscles and travels horizontally forwards to merge with the rectus sheath.

At the side and back of the trunk, the *quadratus lumborum* muscle is also important. It is positioned between the pelvis and ribcage and has an inner and outer portion. The inner

portion is attached directly to the spine and acts to stabilise the spine, while the outer portion has a tendency to get tight and painful during back pain requiring clinical massage treatment (*see* figure 8.1). For further details of trunk muscle structure and function see *The Complete Guide to Abdominal Training* (Norris 2009) published by A&C Black.

## INTERNAL ORGANS (VISCERA)

The abdomen stretches from the lower ribs to the pelvic rim. For descriptive purposes we normally divide it into four quarters (known as *quadrants*) crossing at the umbilicus. The quadrants are named as though your client were describing them themselves, so when you look at them on the bench, their left will be to your right (*see* figure 8.2, which shows the four abdominal quadrants with the major internal organs, or *viscera*, to be found in each).

| Right upper (RU) | Left upper (LU) |
|---|---|
| Liver | Stomach |
| Gallbladder | Spleen |
| Large intestine (colon) | Pancreas |
| Kidney (right) | Kidney (left) |
| Duodenum | Large intestine |
| Small intestine | Small intestine |
| **Right lower (RL)** | **Left lower (LL)** |
| Large intestine | Large intestine |
| Appendix | Small intestine |
| Small intestine | |

**Figure 8.2** The four abdominal quadrants and the major organs found within each

Normal organs are generally not easy to palpate due to their depth beneath the body surface, and it is only when they become enlarged that they become palpable. In very lean subjects the major blood vessel from the heart (the *aorta*) may be seen to pulsate in the abdomen slightly left of the midline.

The liver moves with the diaphragm as you breathe so sometimes the liver can be found on lean subjects at the highest point of the right upper quadrant just beneath the rib when your client breaths in deeply (full inspiration).

### Keypoint

The internal organs (*viscera*) are not easily palpated unless enlarged.

The stomach cannot be palpated unless full, and this becomes even more so when your client is standing or is inhaling deeply, as it then moves down. The large intestine (or *colon*) is made up of a series of sacs and is therefore said to be sacculated. Under deep palpation, firm stool-filled portions may be felt, which are perfectly normal. The small intestine is not saccular, but smooth walled.

## CLASSICAL ABDOMINAL MASSAGE TECHNIQUES

Abdominal massage takes into account the direction of the digestive movements, with the ascending (upwards) colon on the right side of the body, the transverse colon horizontal just beneath the costal margins and the descending (downwards) colon on the left. The aims are to reduce abdominal muscle tension and to induce reflex stimulation of the digestive organs.

The technique is used to relieve pain, bloating and constipation and is both clinically effective and supported by research evidence. A 2009 study (Lamas et al. 2009) compared the success of abdominal massage to that of laxative drugs to reduce constipation in 60 patients. Using a standard research measure (the gastrointestinal symptoms ratings scale, or GSRS, see Svedlund et al. 1988), the study found that the massage group had significantly less symptoms when using abdominal massage and an increase in bowel movements compared to the control group (who were using laxatives only).

## Exercise 8.1 Effleurage

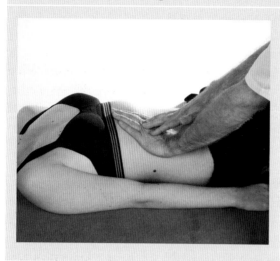

### Purpose

To reduce muscle tension within the abdominals and cause reflex stimulation of the digestive organs.

### Preparation

Begin with your client lying on their back with a pillow under their knees.

### Action

Massage in a clockwise direction using a 'U' shape from pelvis to ribs. Begin on the right-hand side, moving from pelvis to ribs, across the abdomen below the ribs and then downwards from the ribs to the pelvis again.

### Tips

The whole 'U' shaped circuit should take 5–7 seconds.

### Points to note

Vary your hand direction as you move and only use a gentle pressure.

### Exercise 8.2 Petrissage

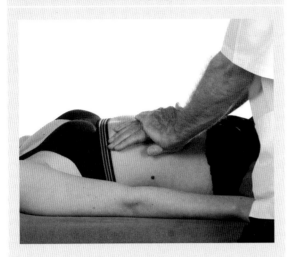

## Purpose

To reduce muscle tension within the superficial abdominal muscles.

## Preparation

Your client should be lying on their back with a roll or pillow beneath their knees. Begin standing side on to your client, with one hand on the side close to you (ipsilateral) the other away from you (contralateral).

## Action

Draw you hands towards each other, applying the petrissage movement with the heel of your hand as you move forwards and your flat fingers as you move backwards. Use a rhythmic movement that targets the whole abdomen from the base of the ribs (costal margin) to the pelvis.

## Tips

Time the massage stroke to the bend of your knees. Sink downwards through your knees and raise again as you move your hands so that the force for the movement comes from your legs.

## Points to note

Tension within the abdomen is common following strenuous training, but may also be due to protective spasm of an underlying medical problem. In cases of persistent abdominal muscle spasm refer your client to a medical doctor.

## Exercise 8.3 Vibrations

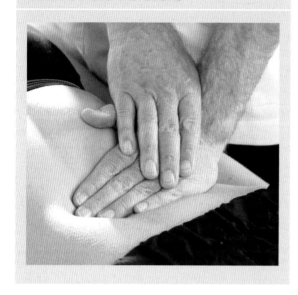

### Purpose
To cause reflex stimulation of the internal organs using light percussion.

### Preparation
Begin with you client lying flat, their legs straight in order to tighten their abdominal region.

### Action
Apply the vibration action using the flat of your hand. Shake your hand for 5–7 seconds in one position before moving to another section of the abdominal wall.

### Tips
To apply a more forceful vibration action use one hand resting on the other.

### Points to note
Percussion techniques such as tapotement (*see* chapter 3, pages 41–2) are generally too powerful for the abdominal region. Vibration/shaking will be better tolerated by your client.

## SPECIALIST CLINICAL MASSAGE TECHNIQUES
We have used classical massage to target the whole abdominal region, and now we shall look at specific clinical massage techniques used to target individual abdominal areas.

**Exercise 8.4** DTF to the intercostals

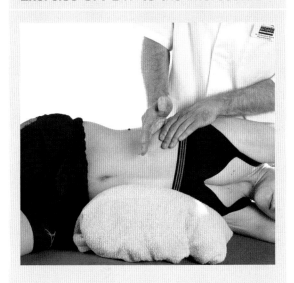

## Purpose

To mobilise the intercostal tissues following extensive rib bruising using deep transverse friction (DTF).

## Preparation

Begin with your client lying on their non-injured side. Lie them flat initially, and then over a pillow to open the ribcage as pain subsides. Use the little finger (ulnar) side of your hand as your massage contact.

## Action

Apply the DTF movement by pressing the side of your hand between the ribs (intercostals space) and then move to and fro along the rib space.

## Tips

First, as the rib is slightly curved your hand movement should follow this. Second, press into the tissues only enough to make a secure contact. Vary your pressure to accommodate to your client's ribcage movements as they breath.

## Points to note

Remember for DTF that your hand and your client's skin move as a single unit to effectively target the tissues beneath. Do not allow your hand to glide over the skin, as the skin friction may cause a burn.

### Exercise 8.5 Intercostal MET using rib fixation

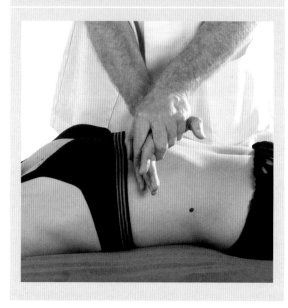

## Purpose
To release tension in the intercostal muscles following rib injury using muscle energy technique (MET).

## Preparation
Begin with your client lying on their back. Locate the area of pain between two adjacent ribs and use the little finger side of your hand as your massage contact. Reach the client's arms overhead to expand the ribcage.

## Action
Press in and down onto the rib below the painful area. Hold this rib fixed using the side of your hand and ask your client to take a deep breath (maximal inspiration) and to hold the in breath for 3–5 seconds. Release and get them to breathe normally for 30 seconds, before repeating.

## Tips
It is important to 'hook' the side of your hand and little finger onto the rib to prevent your hand from slipping over the skin surface, which may cause a friction burn on the skin.

## Points to note
Make sure that your client breaths normally after each maximal inspiration. Breathing deeply too many times can cause hyperventilation and dizziness.

### Exercise 8.6 Pectoralis minor TrP release

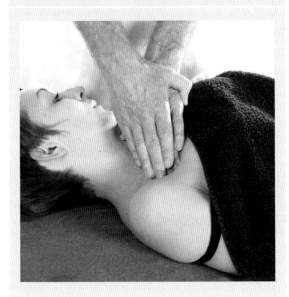

### Purpose

To reduce tension in the pectoralis minor muscle when correcting a shoulder forward posture using trigger point (TrP) release.

### Preparation

Begin with your client lying on their back. When dealing with tightness in the right pectoralis minor, place their left hand over their breast for modesty (and in the opposite direction when treating the left pectoralis).

### Action

Locate the TrP close to the sharp point of bone (known as the corocoid process) within the upper chest in the hollow between the shoulder and outer collar bone (clavicle). Apply gentle pressure, building in strength as pain eases. Hold the point for 30–40 seconds. Follow the TrP release with a passive stretch, fixing your client's upper ribs with one hand and pressing on the front of their shoulder with the other. Hold the stretched position (known as shoulder retraction) for 10–20 seconds.

### Tips

The pectoralis minor muscle assists the breathing action by raising the upper ribs on deep breathing. As you apply the TrP release and muscle stretch, encourage your client to breathe out (exhale) as you apply pressure. The breathing action will help to lower the upper ribs and assist the stretch.

### Points to note

When the pectoralis minor muscle is tight it will tip the scapula forwards. In the lying position, pressure from your client's body weight will help to correct this.

**Exercise 8.7** Diaphragm release

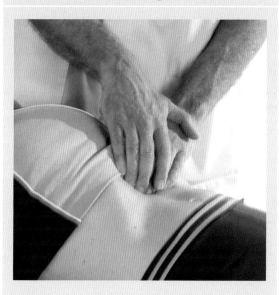

## Purpose

To reduce spasm of the diaphragm in cases of pain or 'stitch'.

## Preparation

Begin with your client sitting propped up on a bench (half-sitting) with their legs bent. Stand behind and slightly to the side of them.

## Action

Place your hands flat over your client's lower ribs with your fingertips resting on their upper abdomen. Gently curl your fingertips around and slightly beneath their lower ribs, sinking in gradually over a period of 20–30 seconds.

## Tips

Apply pressure as your client exhales and their abdomen naturally relaxes. Hold the pressure as they breathe in, but do not press in further.

## Points to note

Once the diaphragm release has been performed, teach your client diaphragmatic breathing. For this, they should allow their abdominal wall to raise (swell) as they inhale and lower (hollow) as they exhale.

## Exercise 8.8 Rectus abdominis insertion, DTM

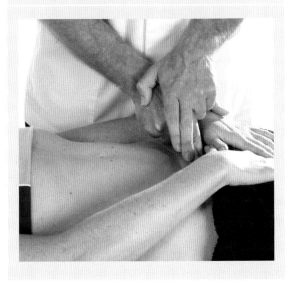

### Purpose
To target the insertion of the rectus abdominis muscle at the pubic bone using deep tissue massage (DTM).

### Preparation
Begin with you client lying flat. For modesty they should place their hand over their genitals. Use your index finger supported by your middle finger as your massage tool.

### Action
Perform DTM to the insertion of the rectus onto the pubic bone from above (so, superiorly). Your hand is held over your client's stomach with your fingers pressing against the top (stomach side) of the pubis.

### Tips
The rectus insertion is normally damaged when performing rapid intensive abdominal training, and as such clients with this condition are normally quite young and fit. Pressure may need to be quite deep and to tighten the tissue, making treatment more effective, place you client's hips up on a block (yoga block) or pillows to move the spine into extension.

### Points to note
Diagnosis is important in this condition, as pubic pain following injury may have a number of causes. Ask a physiotherapist to assess the injury to differentiate muscle injury from disruption of the pubic symphysis and calcification of the pubic tissues (known as osteitis pubis).

**Exercise 8.9** TrP release to iliopsoas

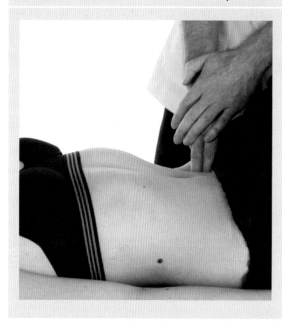

## Purpose

To release pain and tension in the iliopsoas muscle by targeting the trigger point (TrP).

## Preparation

Begin with your client lying flat while you bend your knees and hips. Use the tips of your fingers as your massage contact initially, focusing in on the TrP using your index and middle fingers pressed together.

## Action

Locate the iliopsoas in the lower abdomen lateral to the rectus abdominis muscle. The line of the muscle is diagonal from the lumbar spine to the inner hip (known as the lesser trochanter of the femur). Locate the TrP as a painful nodule or taut band. Apply static compression and hold the tension for 30–60 seconds until the muscle releases.

## Tips

Ask your client to lift their foot 1–2cm from the bench (known as active hip flexion) to tense the iliopsoas, which will make palpation easier.

## Points to note

Once the TrP has released, place the muscle on stretch by putting your client's knee over the bench side to allow the hip to move into extension. Hold the stretched position for 30–60 seconds. Do not allow your client to lift their leg back on to the bench as this will tense the muscle again (known as active hip flexion). Lift their leg for them.

**Exercise 8.10** Frictional massage for bruising over the iliac crest

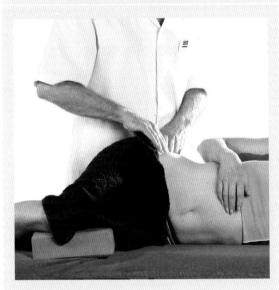

### Purpose
To increase blood flow over the local muscles attaching to the iliac crest following a hip pointer injury.

### Preparation
Begin with your client lying on their unaffected side with their upper hip flexed, knee resting on a pillow. Use your finger pads grasped together or the pisiform (little finger side) region of your hand as your massage contact.

### Action
Perform deep circular frictional massage to increase blood flow. Move into and across the skin region, gradually increasing pressure as your client's discomfort allows.

### Tips
The muscle attachments in the area are quite thick and offer substantial tissue resistance. To produce more power, lower the treatment bench and lean into the massage through straighter arms.

### Points to note
Several muscles attach in this region, including the lateral abdominals (internal and external oblique and transversus), sartorius, tensor fascia lata and rectus femoris. These are injured through direct contact in a hip pointer injury, which may occur through a fall in skiing, or tackle in rugby, for example.

# UPPER LIMB
# // TECHNIQUES

9

## ANATOMY REFRESHER

### BONE AND JOINT STRUCTURES IN THE UPPER LIMBS

The upper limb consists of several bones. The shoulder blade (scapula) is a flat bone lying on the back of the ribcage. At its outer, or lateral, end it narrows into a shallow socket (known as a *glenoid cavity*), which forms a joint with the ball at the top of the upper arm bone (humerus). This joint (*gleno-humeral joint*) is the true shoulder. The scapula is held away from the side of the body by the collar bone (clavicle) which forms a strut.

The clavicle itself forms two joints, one with the scapula, known as the AC or *acromioclavicular* joint, the other with the breastbone (sternum) the SC or *sternoclavicular* joint (*see* figure 9.1).

The AC joint is commonly injured in rugby in a condition called sprung shoulder. The SC joint may be overstretched and inflamed during exercises such as dips or push-ups. Most of the bones are superficial and so easily palpated.

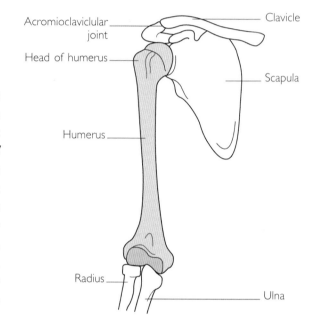

Acromioclaviclular joint
Head of humerus
Humerus
Radius
Clavicle
Scapula
Ulna

**Figure 9.1** The shoulder joints

### MUSCLE STRUCTURES IN THE UPPER LIMBS

The scapula is not fixed to the ribcage but held in place by the balanced pull of muscles attaching to it. On its under surface lies the *subscapularis* muscle, while on the back of the scapula the *supraspinatus* and *infraspinatus* muscles are positioned above and below the scapular spine – a ridge of bone dividing the scapula into two. These small muscles, together with the *teres minor*, form a group called the *rotator cuff* which lies beneath the powerful trapezius muscle spanning from the neck out to the shoulders and back into the centre of the spine.

Although small, the rotator cuff group has an important function, acting as secondary ligaments to hold the ball and socket (glenohumeral) joint together. Because the muscles are very close to the shoulder joint, they are often trapped in it during sport actions, which causes rotator cuff *impingement*. Pain and spasm ensue, and clinical massage is called for to address trigger points and muscle tightness around the area.

As the arm is lifted from the side of the body, the ball in socket joint moves and the scapula slides over the ribcage. Movement of the scapula is controlled by the rhomboid muscles attaching to the inner edge (medial border), the trapezius attaching to the top and bottom (upper and lower trapezius fibres respectively), the levator scapulae attaching to the top of the scapula, and the pectoralis minor attaching to a lip of bone at the front (corocoid process).

Beneath the scapula there are two muscles, the serratus anterior and subscapularis, which hold the bone flat onto the ribcage. These muscles pull together to rotate the scapula upward or downward. Again, they are often involved in postural conditions and injury requiring clinical massage treatment.

## Major muscles of the shoulder region

The major muscles of the shoulder region are the trapezius, latissimus dorsi, pectoralis major and deltoid (*see* figure 9.2).

The *trapezius* has upper fibres which attach to the base of the skull, middle fibres which travel outward to the shoulder (clavicle and spine of the scapula) and the lower fibres move back in again to attach to the middle (thoracic) spine. It is common for the upper trapezius fibres to become tight and painful, requiring clinical massage.

The latissimus dorsi connects the shoulder with the pelvis. Its fibres stretch from the pelvis and sacrum upwards across the lower ribs to attach to the bottom of the scapula (known as the inferior angle) and then into the top of the humerus shaft. The latissimus is involved in lifting actions and its fascial covering is extensive, often becoming tight. Fascial release (FR) techniques for this muscle are very effective in relieving muscular back pain.

The deltoid muscle forms a cap over the shoulder. It has an extensive attachment from the scapula and clavicle and into the outer upper arm (known as the deltoid impression of the humerus). The muscle has anterior, medial and posterior fibres and is often one set of fibres rather than the whole muscle that requires attention when applying clinical massage

At the front of the chest we have the powerful pectoral major muscle with the smaller pectoralis minor lying beneath. The pectoral major is the punching and pressing muscle and as such it is used frequently in daily activities, making it strong and tight. Postural problems often require this muscle to be released in order to correct a round shouldered posture.

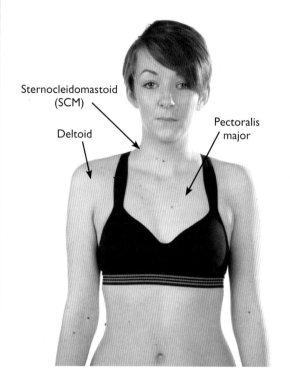
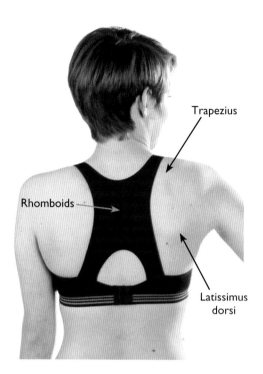

**Figure 9.2** The major muscles of the shoulder region

Several smaller muscles connect from the shoulder to the neck including the sternocleidomastoid (SCM) from the clavicle and sternum to the base of the skull and bone near the ear (which is called the mastoid process) and the levator scapulae from the top of the scapula (known as the superior angle) to the cervical spine. Both muscles if tight will pull the neck out of alignment and commonly encourage the development of deep painful trigger points, which respond to clinical massage techniques.

### Keypoint

The sternocleidomastoid (SCM) and levator scapulae muscles may become tight, pulling the neck out of alignment.

**Exercise 9.1** Latissimus dorsi fascial stretch

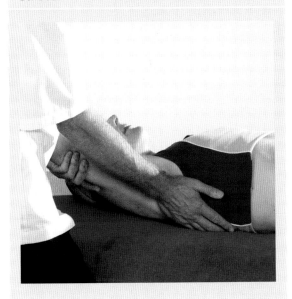

## Purpose

To lengthen the latissimus dorsi muscle and covering fascia.

## Preparation

Begin with your client lying on their back. Stand behind them and raise their right arm over their head, placing it beneath your left arm. Hook your left forearm beneath their arm and press your arm to your side to grip.

## Action

Use your right hand to press onto their shoulder blade (scapula), and at the same time lean back slightly to produce slight traction on their straight arm. Using the heel of your hand as your massage contact, work along the side of the latissimus muscle from the inner arm to their mid-back.

## Tips

Make sure you take a stride stance (*see* page 32) so you can transfer your weight from foot to foot in a rocking action as you press forwards with your hand and then lean back to lengthen their arm.

## Points to note

Some clients find it difficult to lift their arm overhead in a horizontal position. If this is the case, lower the bench and keep the arm slightly forwards as you lift it overhead (which is known as flexion-abduction).

**Exercise 9.2** Subscapularis TrP

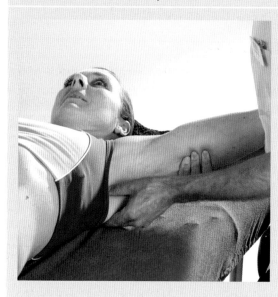

## Purpose
To release tension in the subscapularis muscle on the under-surface of the scapula.

## Preparation
Begin with your client lying on their back. Draw their arm out to 90-degree level (abduction) with the bench. Place your client's arm beneath your right arm, pressing your arm into your side to grip. Lean back slightly to traction (or pull) your client's arm and draw their shoulder blade away from their ribcage. You should be able to see the sharp edge (known as the lateral border) of the shoulder blade pressing through the latissimus dorsi muscle.

## Action
Using your thumb or knuckles as your massage contact, press down onto the exposed edge of the scapula to target the subscapularis.

## Tips
Depending on the size of your client you may need to use a single knuckle or two knuckles pressed together.

## Points to note
The latissimus dorsi is thick in this area, and it is essential to draw the scapula away from the body so that your fingers press onto the under-surface of the scapula. If you do not do this you will press onto the latissimus instead.

**Exercise 9.3** Upper arm DTM in sitting

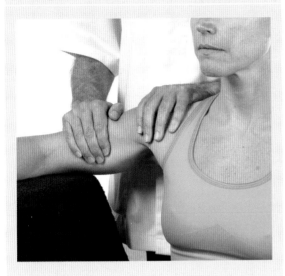

## Purpose
To target the shoulder and upper arm muscles using deep tissue massage (DTM).

## Preparation
Begin with your client sitting in a chair with their arm supported on a table or bench.

## Action
Use the side of your hand (the hypothenar region) as your massage contact. Apply DTM to the lower neck (trapezius), shoulder (deltoid) and upper arm (biceps and triceps) muscles.

## Tips
In this starting position you may move the neck to reposition it, stretch the upper trapezius and rotate the shoulder to access the muscles more easily.

## Points to note
As you are standing above your client and pressing downwards, it is easy to gain a deep pressure. Ensure that the pressure is not painful, however, by getting continuous feedback from your client.

**Exercise 9.4** DTF to biceps long head tendon

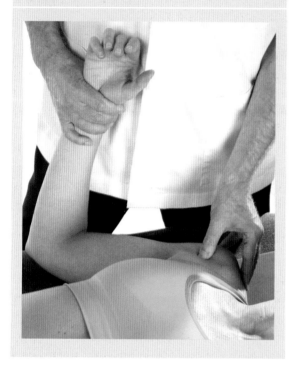

## Purpose

To reduce pain from tendinopathy of the long head of biceps using deep transverse friction (DTF).

## Preparation

Begin with your client lying on a bench with their affected arm bent at the elbow. Use either your thumb pad or one supported finger as your massage contact and place it on the groove at the front of the upper arm bone (known as the bicipital groove of the humerus). Grip your client's forearm with your other hand.

## Action

Keep your finger still, pressing onto the bicipital groove while you turn your client's upper arm (known as humeral rotation) using their forearm as a lever.

## Tips

The biceps tendon lies within the bicipital groove along a length of 2–3cm. Move your finger to different sites until you locate the precise point causing the symptoms.

## Points to note

Remember with DTF that your fingers and your client's skin move as a single unit, so don't allow your fingers to slide over the skin, which can create a friction burn.

**Exercise 9.5** DTF to supraspinatus tendon

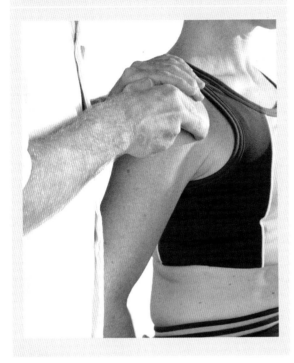

### Purpose
To target the supraspinatus tendon, as it comes onto the front of the shoulder, using deep transverse friction (DTF).

### Preparation
Begin with your client sitting. Place the hand on their injured side behind their back (medial humeral rotation) to tighten the suparspinatus tendon over the front of the shoulder.

### Action
Apply DTF using one finger supported by another. Your direction should be 90 degrees (so transverse) to the tendon that runs parallel to the upper arm bone (humerus).

### Tips
Begin with fairly superficial strokes until the pain begins to ease (which is known as massage analgesia) and then move in more deeply. Apply force in one direction only, pressing deeper as you pull your fingers towards yourself and releasing pressure as you move back. This on-off action will allow your fingers to recover.

### Points to note
Your fingers and your client's skin should move as a single unit – do not slide your fingers across the skin as this can cause friction burn.

**Exercise 9.6** Shoulder rotation, MET

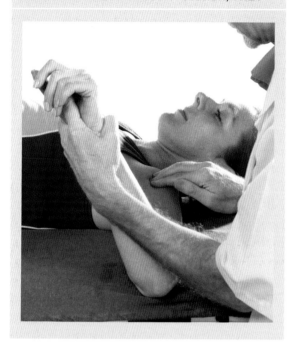

## Purpose

To release tension in the rotator cuff musculature using muscle energy technique (MET).

## Preparation

Begin with your client lying on their back with their shoulder abducted, and elbow flexed to 90 degrees. Their humerus remains supported on the bench. Stabilise their upper arm with one hand and grip their forearm with your other hand.

## Action

Keeping their elbow angle constant, externally rotate your client's humerus, taking their knuckles down towards the bench. Engage the point of resistance and ask them to resist your movement using the instruction 'stop me moving your shoulder'. Hold the tension (through isometric contraction) for 5–10 seconds and then repeat, moving to the new point of resistance.

## Tips

As you grip your client's forearm, control their wrist using your fingers and thumb on their hand.

## Points to note

This action is lateral rotation which stretches the medial rotators of the shoulder (subscapularis, teres major, latissimus dorsi, pectoralis major and anterior deltoid). These muscles have a tendency to tighten in everyday postures, such as sitting at a computer or driving, as these tasks place the shoulder joint into a medially rotated position for prolonged periods.

**Exercise 9.7** Supraspinatus TrP

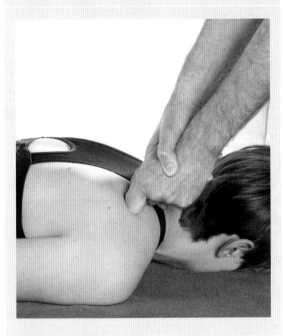

## Purpose

To release pain and tension in the supraspinatus muscle at the upper end of the shoulder blade (scapula).

## Preparation

Begin with your client lying on their painless side. Draw their arm forwards (flexion) and place it on a cushion or block.

## Action

Use one or two knuckles pressed against your thumb as your massage contact. Press into the bulk of the supraspinatus muscle, which lies above the middle ridge of the shoulder blade (spine of the scapula), approximately 8–10cm below the top of the shoulder region.

## Tips

To identify this muscle ask your client to lift their arm from the side of their body (known as abduction) and to swivel their arm outwards (known as lateral rotation) against your resistance. You can identify the muscle by its tensing at the top of the shoulder blade.

## Points to note

Make sure that your pressure is with the flat surface of your finger (or the shaft of the phalanx) rather than your sharp knuckle (known as the interphalangeal joint).

## Exercise 9.8 Infraspinatus TrP

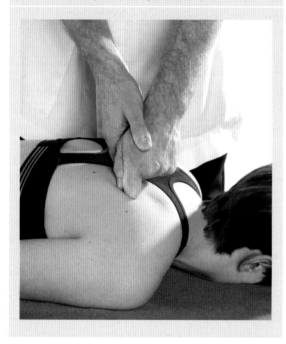

### Purpose
To release pain and tension in the infraspinatus muscle at the lower end of the shoulder blade (scapula).

### Preparation
Begin with your client lying on their front. Draw their arm forwards (known as flexion) and place it on a cushion or block.

### Action
Use one or two knuckles reinforced by your thumb as your massage contact. Press into the bulk of the infraspinatus muscle, which lies below the middle ridge of the shoulder blade (or the spine of the scapula).

### Tips
To identify this muscle ask your client to bend their elbow to 90 degrees and, keeping their upper arm tucked into the side of their body, swivel their arm outwards (lateral rotation) against your resistance. You can identify the muscle as it tenses at the bottom half of shoulder blade.

### Points to note
Make sure that your pressure is with the flat surface of your finger (the shaft of the phalanx) rather than your knuckle (the interphalangeal joint).

**Exercise 9.9** Upper trapezius, DTM in sitting

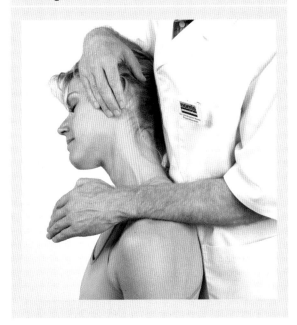

## Purpose
To target the upper fibres of the trapezius muscle using deep tissue massage. (DTM)

## Preparation
Begin with your client sitting upright on a stool or reverse sitting on a chair. Stand behind and to the side of your client using your forearm as your massage contact.

## Action
Place the side of your forearm on the upper and mid trapezius close to the neck. Use a downward and outward (lateral) pressure from the neck to the shoulder (which is called the *acromion process*).

## Tips
If your massage force causes your client to bend sideways, sit them next to your treatment bench and support their opposite arm on the bench.

## Points to note
The action is to massage deeply into the trapezius muscle and at the same time to press the shoulder blade downward and outward.

## Exercise 9.10 Upper trapezius TrP release

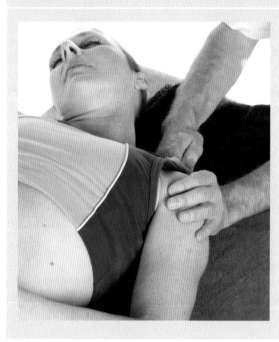

## Purpose

To release an upper trapezius trigger point (TrP).

## Preparation

Begin with your client lying on their back with their head close to the bench end. Side-bend their head away from their painful TrP and hold their head in position with a block or rolled towel. Use one supported knuckle as your massage contact.

## Action

Gently press your supported knuckle into the trapezius muscle using the flat surface of the finger (the shaft of the middle phalanx) rather than the pointed knuckle (the interphalangeal joint). Maintain the pressure for 30–90 seconds, allowing the muscle to release.

## Tips

You may stabilise the shoulder with one hand while applying pressure onto the TrP with the other.

## Points to note

Tipping your client's head to the side tightens the trapezius muscle and makes the TrP release technique more effective.

**Exercise 9.11** Upper trapezius, MET

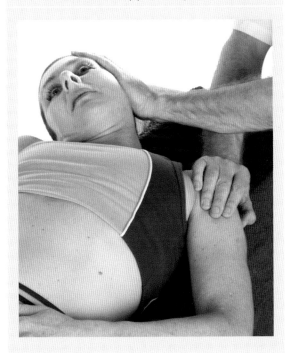

## Purpose
To apply muscle energy technique (MET) to the upper fibres of the trapezius muscle

## Preparation
Begin with your client lying on their back with their head close to the bench end. Side bend their head away from their painful trigger point (TrP). Cross your arms. For pain on the right trapezius, fix your client's neck with your left palm and their shoulder with your right.

## Action
Holding your client's head side bent, gently press downwards on their shoulder (known as scapular depression). Hold the stretched position for 20–30 seconds and then release gradually.

## Tips
To enhance the stretch, apply pressure as your client is breathing out (exhaling).

## Points to note
The pressure is to the shoulder, not the delicate neck structures. The right hand maintains neck position, but does not push into further side-bending. Rest the elbow of your couch-level arm on a folded towel for support.

### Exercise 9.12 Pectoralis major, MET in lying

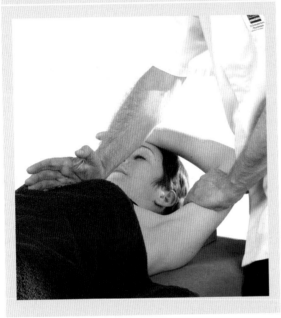

## Purpose

To lengthen the pectoralis major muscle using muscle energy technique (MET).

## Preparation

Begin with your client lying with the shoulder and elbow of the affected arm flexed, and the back of the hand placed on their forehead. Stand to the side of your client and stabilise their shoulder with your close arm. Grip their upper arm with your far hand and press their elbow backwards and downwards (abduction and extension, respectively) until the point of resistance is engaged.

## Action

Ask your client to perform an isometric contraction of the pectoralis using the instruction 'don't let me move your arm any further'. Hold the contraction for 5–10 seconds and then relax. Move to the new resistance point and repeat.

## Tips

Take care not to press onto the inner aspect of your client's shoulder as the ulnar nerve is fairly superficial here and direct pressure may be painful.

## Points to note

This technique targets the sternal fibres of the pectoralis major. The clavicular fibres are stretched using less shoulder abduction but more extension (so you would need to get the client's arm to brush the side of the body).

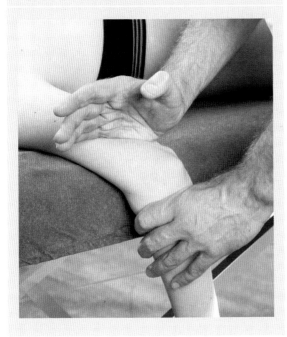

**Exercise 9.13** Triceps insertion, DTM

## Purpose

To target the triceps muscle insertion on the back of the elbow using deep tissue massage (DTM).

## Preparation

Begin with your client lying on their front with their upper arm supported on the bench and elbow bent to 90 degrees. Use the little finger side of your hand (the hypothenar eminence) as your massage contact.

## Action

Target the triceps muscle attachment between the point of the elbow (the olecranon process) and the upper arm bone (the humerus). Use gradually increasing pressure directed downwards and across the tendon to impart compression and shearing forces to the tissues.

## Tips

To apply additional shearing force and create a fascial release (FR), lock the tissues and have your client bend and straighten their arm.

## Points to note

Do not press directly over the point of the elbow as this will be painful.

## Exercise 9.14 DTF to the common extensor origin

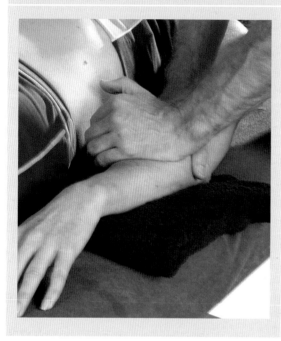

### Purpose

To treat the common extensor origin in cases of tennis elbow (medical name extensor tendinopathy) using deep transverse friction (DTF).

### Preparation

Begin with your client sitting with their forearm supported on a block or folded towel. Their wrist and elbow should be bent (flexed) in order to tighten the forearm extensor muscles. Your massage contact is your index finger supported by your middle finger, slightly curved and pressed together, or the side of your hand.

### Action

Press into your client's skin over the tight area and perform the DTF, avoiding moving across the skin surface as this will cause friction burn. Aim to move the tissues by 1–2cm, maintaining the depth of the action and pressing into the tissues.

### Tips

Press into the tissues harder as you pull your fingers towards yourself and release pressure on the recovery stroke to allow your fingers to rest.

### Points to note

As the massaged area becomes numb (known as massage analgesia) you are able to press more deeply.

## Exercise 9.15 Forearm extensor, MET in sitting

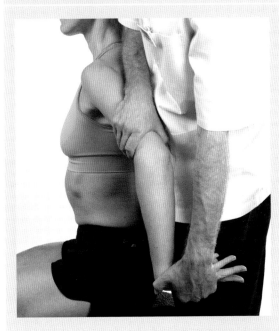

### Purpose
To reduce tension in the forearm extensor muscles in cases of tennis elbow using muscle energy technique (MET).

### Preparation
Begin with your client sitting. Stand behind them and take their arm backwards (into shoulder extension), keeping the elbow unlocked. Flex the wrist (palm to forearm) and pronate the forearm, taking the thumb away from the body.

### Action
Flex your client's wrist maximally and gradually extend their elbow to the point of resistance or mild pain. Stop at the onset of this point (do not press into it) and ask your client to try to extend their wrist against your resistance (known as isometric contraction). Hold this tension for 5–10 seconds and then release. Keep the wrist fully flexed and extend the elbow to the new point of resistance/pain and repeat.

### Tips
Make sure you do not put your thumb into the wrist crease as this will block full wrist flexion.

### Points to note
This position is used by physiotherapists in a soft tissue manipulation (high velocity thrust) called Mill's procedure. The technique described above should remain as a stretch, however, with no thrust being applied.

**Exercise 9.16** Forearm flexor, DTM

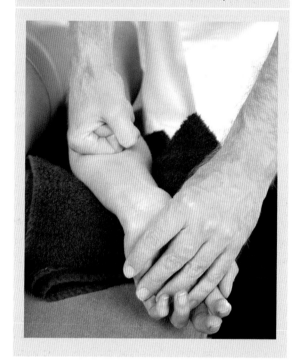

## Purpose

To release tension within the forearm flexor muscles using deep tissue massage. (DTM)

## Preparation

Begin with your client lying on a bench with their arm held loosely from their side (abducted) and forearm placed on a folded towel. Use your loose fist as your massage contact.

## Action

Stabilise your client's forearm with one hand and apply compression using the flat of your fist. Gradually move up the forearm from the wrist, increasing pressure as the tissues become thicker.

## Tips

If your fist is considerably wider than your client's forearm, restrict your contact to the index and middle fingers only.

## Points to note

The forearm flexor muscles are often worked much harder than the extensors in manual activities in both work and sport. Tension in the muscles leading to pain, cramping and reduced blood flow (medical name ischaemia) is common. DTM is an effective method of managing this condition.

## Exercise 9.17 DTF to common flexor origin

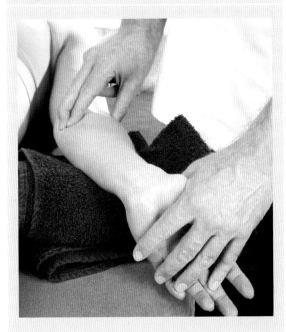

### Purpose
To release the flexor tendon attachment using deep transverse friction (DTF).

### Preparation
Begin with your client lying with their arms by their side, forearms turned palm upwards. Use your index and middle fingers pressed together and slightly bent (flexed) as your massage contact.

### Action
Perform the DTF sweeping across the tendon tissue attaching to the knobble of bone on the inner aspect of your client's elbow (known as the medial epicondyle). Apply pressure on the upward stroke, relaxing slightly and allowing your fingers to recover on the downward stroke.

### Tips
To stretch the tendons while applying the DTF, have your client place their hand clear of the edge of the bench. Draw their wrist backwards (into extension) and hold their hand in this position with your other hand or using pressure from your leg.

### Points to note
As the tissue area becomes numb (known as massage analgesia) you may apply a more forceful massage.

**Exercise 9.18** Tennis elbow TrPs

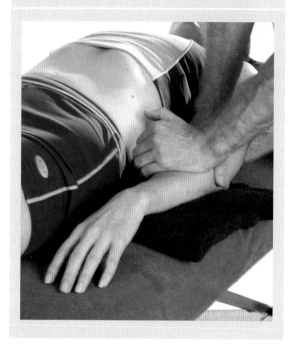

### Purpose
To release trigger points (TrPs) within the forearm extensor muscles (extensor carpi radialis longus and brevis).

### Preparation
Begin with your client lying on their back, with their forearm supported on a folded towel or resting on the bench. Use the angle of your wrist on the little finger side (pisiform bone) or two knuckles as your massage contact.

### Action
Press into the forearm extensor muscles, moving from the elbow to the lower forearm. Localise pressure on any nodules or tight tissue bands found. Hold the pressure for 30–90 seconds on each painful area until pain subsides.

### Tips
To tighten the extensor muscles, bend (flex) your client's wrist over the edge of the bench.

### Points to note
The longer forearm extensor muscle (extensor carpi radialis longus) attaches slightly above the elbow, so continue your massage above the elbow crease where pain is found in this region.

## Exercise 9.19 Tennis elbow acupressure massage

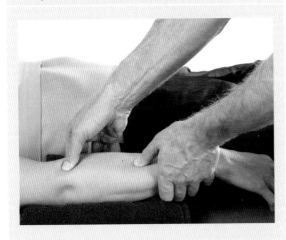

### Purpose

To relieve pain from tennis elbow using acupuncture points.

### Preparation

Begin by locating acupuncture points along the large intestine (LI) meridian. Points LI-11, LI-10, and LI-4 may be used. LI-11 is located at the end of the elbow crease when the elbow is maximally bent (flexed), LI-10 lies two thumb breadths below this point on the meridian line to the thumb. L1-4 is found at the thickest part of the thumb muscle (adductor pollicis) when the thumb and forefinger are pressed together (*see* figure 9.3).

### Action

Using your thumbs or index and middle fingers pressed together as your massage contact, apply pressure to each acupuncture point in turn. Build pressure gradually and hold for 10–20 seconds. Repeat the action three times.

### Tips

Apply pressure along the meridian line LI-11, LI-10, LI-4 rather than in a haphazard way.

### Points to note

LI-4 is a very powerful acupuncture point and it is common for your client to feel a deep aching sensation spreading into their thumb when manipulating this point. This sensation is called deqi in traditional Chinese acupuncture practice and is said to represent the arrival of healing qi energy into the area. It is known as *sensory propagation* along the channel in Western medicine.

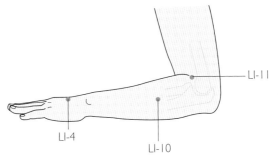

**Figure 9.3** Acupuncture points along the large intestine (LI) meridian.

### Exercise 9.20 Thumb tendon, DTM

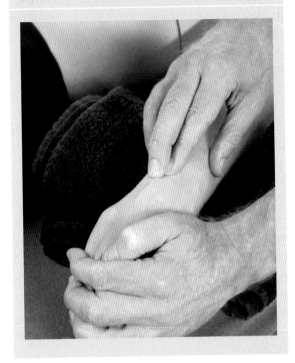

## Purpose

To reduce pain in the thumb tendons at the angle of the wrist using deep tissue massage (DTM).

## Preparation

Begin with the little finger side (ulnar) of your client's forearm resting on a folded towel. Bend their wrist downward (known as ulnar deviation) to stretch the thumb tendons. Use your index finger reinforced by your middle finger as your massage contact.

## Action

Massage along the lower forearm and thumb either side of the wrist bone (known as the ulnar styloid) using circular frictions. Apply deep local effleurage (*see* page 38) along the tendon sheaths.

## Tips

Take the tip of your client's thumb to the base of their little finger to increase the thumb tendon stretch.

## Points to note

This area may be inflamed as well as painful in a condition called De Quervain's tenosynovitis. Where pain does not resolve with clinical massage alone, refer your client to a physiotherapist.

**Exercise 9.21** Wrist extensor, STR

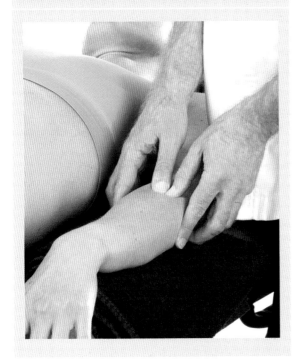

## Purpose

To release tension in the extensor fascia over the back of the forearm using soft tissue release (STR).

## Preparation

Begin with your client's forearm resting on the bench with their wrist at the bench edge. Have them lift up (extend) their wrist. Use your two thumbs pressed together to reinforce them as your massage contact.

## Action

Apply a tissue lock by pressing your thumbs into the extensor muscles close to your client's elbow. Maintain the lock and ask your client to bend their wrist downwards (or to flex) over the bench edge. Release the lock and reapply to the adjacent tissues.

## Tips

The action is to press downwards and towards your client's elbow to impart a shearing force into the forearm tissues.

## Points to note

Your pressure should be firm but not painful.

**Exercise 9.22** Wrist flexor
retinaculum tissue stretch

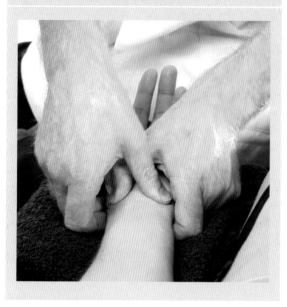

## Purpose

To release tension in the flexor retinaculum across
the wrist.

## Preparation

Begin with your client's wrist and forearm palm
upwards, supported on a folded towel. Your
massage contact is through two thumbs or the
index and middle finger combined on each hand.

## Action

Apply pressure over the wrist bones (the carpals)
on the inside (ulnar) and outside (radial) aspect
of the wrist. Build the pressure slowly and hold
the stretch for 10–20 seconds.

## Tips

Pressure should be angled downwards and
outwards from the centre of the wrist.

## Points to note

The flexor retinaculum can become tight in a
condition called carpal tunnel syndrome. The
tightness and tissue swelling beneath presses on
the medial nerve, sending pain and tingling into
the hand. The clinical massage stretch described
can be used to relieve symptoms when they are
mild. If symptoms continue, refer your client to
a physiotherapist.

## Exercise 9.23 Hand tendon, DTM

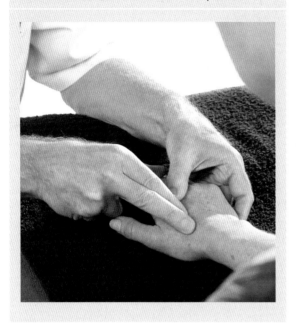

### Action
Use direct pressure, circular frictional massage and local effleurage between the hand bones (the metacarpals).

### Tips
To alter emphasis, place your client's hand over a tennis ball to draw the hand bones apart as you massage.

### Points to note
Encourage your client to perform finger abduction exercises, keeping the fingers straight and moving them apart and together between treatment sessions. This will prevent the swelling from building up again.

### Purpose
To mobilise the soft tissues between the fingers following bruising and swelling using deep tissue massage (DTM).

### Preparation
Begin with your client sitting in a chair, hand flat on a treatment bench. Sit opposite them and use you index finger supported by your middle finger as your massage contact.

### Summary of key terms

- **Analgesia** Pain relieving
- **De Quervain's tenosynovitis** Painful swelling of the thumb tendon sheaths caused by repeated thumb movements, usually made in the workplace
- **Flexor retinaculum** Broad tissue stretching across the underside of the wrist
- **Tendinopathy** Painful condition affecting a tendon

# CLINICAL MASSAGE // RESEARCH

10

Clinical massage therapy is a combination of art and science. The intuitive use of massage, using what 'feels right', must be balanced with the scientific proof that the techniques achieve what therapists claim they do. This process of *evidence-based practice (EBP)* is important if clinical massage is to become more widely accepted within the general medical world. EBP means combining your own clinical knowledge and experience (expertise) with that of the best available science in terms of research papers, tracking your patient results (through clinical audit) and using textbooks (to give a basis in science). Clinical massage quickly becomes out of date unless new knowledge is gained. This knowledge comes from studying your own clinical experience (known as clinical reflection), continuing learning by attending new courses and reading books and research papers. In this chapter we will take a look at some of the research underlying clinical massage in an attempt to strengthen its evidence base.

## STUDIES IN PAIN

Clients often seek clinical massage therapy to reduce pain, and pain research has been used extensively to study the effects of massage. Two major mechanisms for the effect of massage on pain have been proposed. The first is closure of the *pain gate* (a mechanism where a nerve stimulus such as that produced by massage is able to cancel out the feeling of pain) the second is the reduction in *substance P* (*see* 'Definition' box).

### Definition

*Substance P* is a neuropeptide (nerve chemical) involved in the transmission of pain into the central nervous system (CNS). It is released by sensory nerve fibres in the soft tissues and joints as part of the process of inflammation.

Massage will act as a counterirritant, with the sensory stimulus from massage blocking that of the pain at the level of the spinal cord, effectively closing the pain gate. Massage may also enhance deep sleep and through this reduce the amount of substance P which is produced, by allowing the body time to recover.

## STUDIES IN LOW BACK PAIN

In a study looking at low back pain Hernandez-Reif et al. (2000) compared massage therapy with relaxation in 24 subjects. The massage therapy group received classical massage techniques on the back and legs, while the relaxation group received 30 minutes of progressive muscle relaxation, each over a five-week period. The massage therapy group showed a better mood improvement score (based on the profile of mood states depression scale, or the POMS-D – *see* 'Definition' box), less pain (based on the visual analogue scale, or the VAS – *see* 'Definition' box) and an increased range of motion to trunk flexion (angle in degrees) compared to the relaxation group. In addition the massage group showed less sleep disturbance, an important factor as loss of sleep is a common complaint in clients who suffer from low back pain. Blood levels of both serotonin and dopamine (*see* chapter 1) were increased in the massage therapy group.

### Definition

The POMS-D is a shortened form (subscale) of the profile of mood states questionnaire which consists of 65 descriptive words (adjectives). Clients tick the adjectives that they feel best apply to them and come up with a personal score reflecting mood states that include anxiety, depression and anger.

### Definition

A *visual analogue scale* (VAS) is a linear (straight line) scale used in psychometric testing. When used for pain it is normally recorded as a millimetre (mm) measure from 0 (no pain) to 100 (maximum pain). See below for further information and an example of a VAS that you can use with your own clients.

## STUDIES IN FIBROMYALGIA

In a group of 30 patients suffering from fibromyalgia Field et al. (2002) looked at pain and substance P levels. Three groups were used: massage, transcutaneous nerve stimulation or TENS (an electrical stimulation treatment used to deaden pain) and a control group who were given a sham treatment (non-functioning TENS). Each was given a twice weekly treatment over a five-week period. The massage therapy group showed decreased depression, improved sleep (hours), decreased pain (on the VAS scale and in the lower number of tender points) and reduced substance P when compared to the other groups.

## STUDIES IN SHORT-TERM PAIN RELIEF

Looking at short-term pain relief, Seers et al. (2008) conducted a randomised controlled trial (RCT) of a single application of massage therapy to 101 patients with chronic pain. The subjects were split into two groups: intervention (this group was treated with massage) and control (this group was treated with non-massage). The massage therapy group received a 15-minute massage to the back, neck and shoulders while the control group received a 15-minute discussion about their pain. Pain was assessed using the VAS scale and using a *McGill Pain Questionnaire* (*see* 'Definition' box). Pain score on the VAS scale for the massage group was 57.7 after treatment while that for the control group 62.3. The McGill rating was 27.3 and 25.1 respectively.

### Definition

The *McGill Pain Questionnaire* (or the McGill Pain Index) is a standardised rating scale developed at McGill University. It consists of 20 batches of words used to describe pain, and patients circle the terms which they feel best describe their pain. See table 10.1 opposite for an example of a shortened McGill Pain Questionnaire that you can use with your own clients.

## RECORDING CHANGES IN PAIN IN YOUR OWN CLIENTS

Rating and recording changes in pain before and after clinical massage therapy is an important indicator of improvement in your client's condition. Both a VAS scale and pain questionnaire should be use, as they give different types of information.

### The VAS scale

A VAS scale is a quickly applied 'ballpark' figure which you can question your client about throughout treatment to assess tissue irritability (*see* page 64). Rather than asking if a technique is making your client's pain better, rate the scale from one to ten prior to treatment and record changes throughout treatment. Figure 10.1 shows an example of a VAS scale as used in hospital physiotherapy departments within the National Health Service (NHS).

### Pain questionnaires

A pain questionnaire gives a much broader view of the type of pain experienced, and indicates whether pain is changing in nature rather than simply intensity. Table 10.1 shows a short example of the standard McGill form adapted for use in the day-to-day clinical environment. Different aspects of the questionnaire represent different types of description used in pain research (sensory, affective and evaluative). The client circles *seven* terms which best describe their pain: (i) *three* words in groups 1–10, (ii) *two* words in groups 11–15, (iii) *one* word in group 16, and (iv) *one* word in groups 17–20. The points (which derive from the group number in which the word is circled) are then added to give a total score.

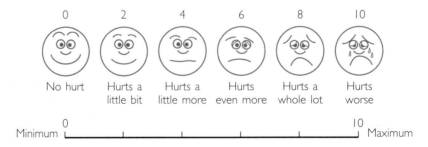

**Figure 10.1** The VAS scale

| Table 10.1 | An adapted form of the McGill Questionnaire |
| --- | --- |
| **Group** | **Descriptive words for the pain** |
| 1 | Flickering, Pulsing, Quivering, Throbbing, Beating, Pounding |
| 2 | Jumping, Flashing, Shooting |
| 3 | Pricking, Boring, Drilling, Stabbing |
| 4 | Sharp, Cutting, Lacerating |
| 5 | Pinching, Pressing, Gnawing, Cramping, Crushing |
| 6 | Tugging, Pulling, Wrenching |
| 7 | Hot, Burning, Scalding, Searing |
| 8 | Tingling, Itchy, Smarting, Stinging |
| 9 | Dull, Sore, Hurting, Aching, Heavy |
| 10 | Tender, Taut (tight), Rasping, Splitting |
| 11 | Tiring, Exhausting |
| 12 | Sickening, Suffocating |
| 13 | Fearful, Frightful, Terrifying |
| 14 | Punishing, Gruelling, Cruel, Vicious, Killing |
| 15 | Wretched, Blinding |
| 16 | Annoying, Troublesome, Miserable, Intense, Unbearable |
| 17 | Spreading, Radiating, Penetrating, Piercing |
| 18 | Tight, Numb, Squeezing, Drawing, Tearing |
| 19 | Cool, Cold, Freezing |
| 20 | Nagging, Nauseating, Agonising, Dreadful, Torturing |

# STUDIES IN IMMUNITY

Immunity to disease is obviously important to all, but from a clinical massage perspective two areas are of interest. The first is the temporary suppression of immunity, which occurs following intense bouts of exercise, such as long distance running and heavy weight training. Here we see an increased risk of upper respiratory tract (nose and throat) infections which often hampers competitive athletes. The second area of interest is with chronic diseases such as HIV and cancer where the immune system is compromised due to the disease itself or to treatments such as radiotherapy and chemotherapy in cancer care. Again there is an increased risk of infection, but with a compromised immune system, relatively light infections can become life threatening. If we can show that massage enhances the body's natural immunity, we can argue for its continued use in the management of all of these conditions.

## STUDIES INTO HIV INFECTION

Diego et al. (2001) looked at the effect of massage on patients with HIV infection. They monitored immunity using the disease markers CD4 and the ratio of CD4/CD8, as well as the number of natural killer (NK) cells in the blood. The CD (standing for *cluster of differentiation*) substances are glycoproteins, which essentially act as receptors on the wall of white blood cells, while NK cells are a type of white blood cell important for immunity. Twenty-four patients with HIV were treated in the study and either received a 20-minute chair massage or the equivalent in relaxation therapy without massage. Questionnaires to assess anxiety and mood showed that while both groups decreased in anxiety, only the massage group reduced in depression. There was an increase in both CD4 count and CD4/CD8 ratio in the massage group alone. NK cell number also increased significantly in the massage group only.

## STUDIES IN LEUKAEMIA

In a similar study the results were repeated in children with leukaemia (Field et al. 2001). Two groups were formed (n=20) with one group (the intervention group) receiving massage and the other (the control group) not receiving massage. The massage group showed less anxiety and depression compared to the control group, and blood measures of immunity (white blood count, neutrophil number and haemoglobin level) all increased in the massage group alone (*see* figure 10.2).

## STUDIES IN TISSUE EFFECTS

Massage is assumed to have a number of tissue effects (*see* chapter 1) but we need to look at the hard evidence to back up these claims. Massage is often claimed to produce heating effects useful in a warm-up for sport, or to warm tissues prior to stretching. Looking at back massage in normal subjects, Longworth (1982) reported increased skin temperature following 6 minutes of effleurage massage, but this tissue temperature increase dropped back to prior massage levels (baseline) within only 10 minutes, suggesting that any benefits will only be available within the treatment period.

Even though the skin becomes red and its temperature raises, does this necessarily affect the soft tissues beneath? In a study which looked at temperature changes in both the skin and subcutaneous tissues (at depths of 1.5, 2.5 and

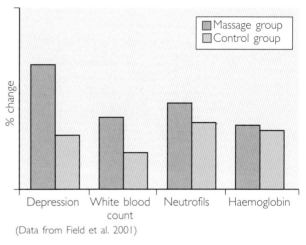

(Data from Field et al. 2001)

**Figure 10.2** Changes in immune function following clinical massage

3.5cm), Drust et al. (2003) used effleurage on the vastus lateralis (outer quadriceps muscle) in seven healthy males, and this treatment showed significant temperature increases. However, the temperature rise went only to a depth of 2.5cm, not to 3.5cm, so changes are very superficial using this massage technique. Although blood flow to the local microcirculation (small blood vessels) may change, regional blood flow (to larger areas) remains largely unchanged (Weerapong et al. 2005).

Reduction in muscle tension is often detected clinically, and scientific evidence does support this. Measuring the H-reflex (*Hoffman reflex*, *see* 'Definition' box) Morelli et al. (1990) used petrissage massage for a maximum of 6 minutes and showed reduced H-reflex activity (known as amplitude) during massage. This returned to baseline when massage stopped, but this study suggests a useful method to relax muscle tone during treatment to facilitate other techniques such as stretching.

### Definition

The *Hoffman reflex*, or H-reflex, is an electrically induced twitch measured using an EMG machine (electromyograph). It is used in muscle studies as a controlled version of the stretch reflex, which it mimics.

### Summary of key terms

- **Counterirritant** Stimulus which distracts a client from their pain
- **Fibromyalgia** Medical condition characterised by widespread pain and altered sensation. Symptoms also often include fatigue, joint pain, and sleep disturbance.
- **Leukaemia** Cancer of the blood or bone marrow.
- **Progressive muscle relaxation** Relaxation method involving tensing and then relaxing muscle groups in a sequence throughout the body.

Looking at hamstring flexibility measured using the straight leg raise (SLR) action, Hopper et al. (2005) showed short-term benefits in movement range after 8 minutes of massage in a group of 35 hockey players. Two groups were formed, using either classical massage or dynamic (active) soft tissue release (STR). Statistically, significant increases in passive motion range were noted in both groups, but movement range returned to baseline within 24 hours, demonstrating a limited immediate effect of clinical massage on hamstring flexibility.

Interestingly this study showed a superior effect of active STR when measured by passive knee extension (hip fixed, knee moving only), but not with passive straight leg raise (movement at both hip and knee), perhaps indicating a greater clinical massage effect on the lower portion of the hamstrings.

# GLOSSARY

**Anticoagulants** Chemical which stops blood clotting

**Beating** Striking the skin with the side of the open fist, also known as pounding

**Blood perfusion** Allowing the muscles to relax and recover between massage strokes, which allows fresh blood to enter the area

**Bony landmarks** Distinguishing features found on the bones of the skeletal system – anything from a line or a notch in its surface to a large bump or projection

**Brushing** Light fingertip pressure used to end a massage and maintain a feeling of relaxation

**Bursa** Small fluid-filled sac that provides a cushion between bones and tendons and/or muscles around a joint, thereby helping to reduce friction between the bones and allowing freedom of movement

**Chopping** Striking the skin with the sides of your hands

**Chronic** Longer term pain

**Clinical reasoning (CR)** Methodical approach to deciding which treatments are appropriate, when they should be used and why

**Compression force** Pressing force that can be applied rapidly with a tapping or cupping force or slowly with a petrissage (pressure) movement. Where a compressive force is applied using a small contact area, such as a fingertip, the effect on tissue is more marked than when the same force is applied using a broader area, such as the palm.

**Connective tissue** Generalised body material made up of cells, fibres and ground substance

**Contraindications** Conditions a client may have which make clinical massage unsuitable

**Contralateral** Pertaining to, situated on, or affecting the opposite side

**Cortisol** Hormone produced by the adrenal glands, which are located on top of the kidneys

**Counterirritant** Stimulus which distracts a client from their pain

**Cutaneous** Of the skin

**Cytoskeleton** Cellular skeleton contained within a cell's cytoplasm and formed out of protein

**Disorganised tissue** Destruction of an organ or tissue or its haphazard form when it heals, with fibres pointing in every direction

**Distal** Anatomically located far from a point of reference, such as an origin or a point of attachment

**Dopamine** A nerve chemical produced in the brain

**Dorsiflexion** The movement which decreases the angle between the dorsum (superior surface) of the foot and the leg, so that the toes are brought closer to the shin, for example

**Extracellular region** Outside of the cell

**Fascia** Thin fibrous membrane which surrounds other tissues such as muscles and ligaments, linking them together

**Fibrin** Blood chemical involved in clotting

**Grip** Holding the tissues to manipulate them

**Hyperflexible** Describes a joint that bends more than the average

**Hysteresis** Property of tissue that enables it to give way or pay out under a constant force

**Inner range** From a position halfway through the full range to a position where the muscle is fully shortened

**Intercellular region** Inside of the cell

**Ipsilateral** Affecting the same side of the body

**Isometric contraction** Where a muscle is contracted against resistance

**Lateral flexion** A movement away from the midline of the body

**Locked** When the fascia is fixed at one point

**Lateral movement** Movement across a bench in line with the short edge

**Longitudinal movement** Movement in line with the long side edge of a treatment bench

**Massage analgesia** Massage that causes the tissue area to become numb, thereby reducing pain

**Myofibroblasts** A cell that is in between a fibroblast and a smooth muscle cell in differentiation

**Neoplasm** Tumour or any new and/or abnormal cell growth

**Oedema** Medical term for swelling

**Organised** Tissue fibres that align in the strongest direction

**Osteoblasts** Cells responsible for bone formation

**Outer range** From a position where the muscle is on full stretch to a position halfway through the full range

**Pain pathway** Pathways leading to and from the brain that inform the brain of the pain and modulate it in response

**Petrissage** Lifting and rolling or wringing actions which are performed by lightly gripping (compressing) the skin

**Plantarflexion** Movement which increases the approximate 90 degree angle between the front part of the foot and the shin, for example

**Protracted** When a muscle is extended forward

**Proximal** Nearest to a point of reference, as to a centre or median line or to the point of attachment or origin

**Regeneration** When tissue regrowth begins

**Remodelling** Healing of injured tissue taking place specifically during the chronic phase, the final stage on the healing timescale, and lasting from 21 days onwards

**Repetitive strain injuries (RSI)** Injury of the musculoskeletal and nervous systems that may be caused by repetitive tasks, forceful exertions, vibrations, mechanical compression (pressing against hard surfaces), sustained or awkward positions

**Screw home effect** Action when the knee reaches full extension. Just as it locks into extension it rotates several degrees in an outward direction, which has the effect of placing most of the weight onto the cartilage, menisci and bones of the joint, resting the thigh and calf muscles

**Selective tissue tension** Examining tissues by stressing to different degrees

**Sensory nerve endings** Sensors within the skin which are responsible for feeling

**Sensory perception** Conscious mental registration of a sensory stimulus (such as pain)

**Sesamoid** Small bone embedded within a tendon which passes close to a joint. It protects the tendon and acts as a pivot point increasing the leverage effect (mechanical advantage) of the tendon.

**Shear force** Occurs when the force is applied at an angle to the tissue, which creates a combination of both compression and stretch

**Slip** Sliding across the tissues to stimulate them

**Static stretch** Tension applied to the muscle

**Stride standing** Massage stance with wide legs, used when facing the side of the bench for lateral movements or short-range longitudinal actions

**Stripping** Deep stroking action a little like firm local effleurage

**Synapse** Junction between two nerve cells, consisting of a minute gap across which impulses pass by diffusion of a neurotransmitter.

**Tactile feedback** Ability of the physiotherapist to feel changes in the joints

**Tapotement** Variety of striking actions which are used to stimulate blood flow to the tissues

**Tapping** Striking the skin with your fingertips

**Tension force** Occurs when two ends of a structure are pulled apart. Sustained tension causes tissues to elongate.

**Thixotropy** Property of certain materials which are normally quite stiff (they have high viscosity) to become more fluid and flow (to have low viscosity) when agitated or subjected to physical stress

**Thousand hands** Massage technique that involves drawing one hand across the body surface towards you (heel of the hand to fingers) and just as the fingertips are about to leave the skin, the heel of the other hand contacts the skin. The feeling is one of a continuous skin stimulation.

**Torsion force** Used in wringing actions where the hands are gripping the client's tissues and turning in opposite directions. Torsion stretches the tissue in a rotary manner and may be used to enhance tissue pliability.

**Trigger point** Painful point in the muscle that can be felt as a nodule or band

**Triple response** Response in the skin which shows as a red, slightly raised area as the blood flow increases during skin stimulation

**Twitch response** When a muscle jumps from sudden pressure or flicking of the fingers across the trigger point band within that muscle, also known as a jump sign

**Vasodilation** When blood vessels open

**Venous return** Rate of blood flow back to the heart

**Viscera** Internal organs

**Viscosity** Describes a fluid's internal resistance to flow, for example water is thinner and less viscous while honey is thicker and more viscous

**Walk standing** Massage stance with one foot a step forwards, used when facing the top or bottom of the bench to give longitudinal movements

**Weal** Minor swelling

# REFERENCES

Brummitt, J. (2008), 'The role of massage in sports performance and rehabilitation: Current evidence and future direction', *North American Journal of Sports Physical Therapy*, 3(1): 7–21.

Cafarelli, E., Sim, J., Carolan, B. and Liebesman, J. (1990), 'Vibratory massage and short-term recovery from muscular fatigue', *International Journal of Sports Medicine*, Dec 11(6): 474–478.

Cromie, J. E., Robertson, V. J. and Best, M. O. (2000), 'Work-related musculoskeletal disorders in physical therapists: Prevalence, severity, risks, and responses', *Physical Therapy*, April 80(4): 336–351.

CSP (2005), *Work-related musculoskeletal disorders affecting members of the Chartered Society of Physiotherapy* (Chartered Society of Physiotherapy, London).

CSP (2004), *Consent: Briefing paper PA 60* (Chartered Society of Physiotherapy, London).

Cyriax, J. (1944), *Deep Massage and Manipulation* (Bailliere Tindall, London).

Diego, M., Field, T. and Hernandez-Reif, M. (2001), 'HIV adolescents show improved immune function following massage therapy', *International Journal of Neuroscience*, 106: 35–45.

Drust, B., Atkinson, G. and Gregson, W. (2003), 'The effects of massage on intramuscular temperature in the vastus lateralis in humans', *International Journal of Sports Medicine*, 24(6): 395–399.

Field, T. (2006), *Massage Therapy Research* (Elsevier, Oxford).

Field, T., Cullen, C. and Diego, M. (2001), 'Leukemia immune changes following massage therapy', *Journal of Bodywork and Movement Therapies*, 5: 271–274.

Field, T., Diego, M. and Cullen, C. (2002), 'Fibromyalgia pain and substance P decrease and sleep improves after massage therapy', *Journal of Clinical Rheumatology*, 8: 72–76.

Gaskell, L. (2008), 'Musculoskeletal assessment'. In Porter, S. (ed.), *Tidy's Physiotherapy* (Churchill Livingstone, Edinburgh).

Goodall-Copestake, B. (1926), *The Theory and Practice of Massage* (Lewis, London).

Graham, D. (1884), *Practical Treatise on Massage* (Wood, New York).

Hernandez-Reif, M., Field, T. and Krasnegor, J. (2000), 'Lower back pain is reduced and range of motion increased after massage therapy', *International Journal of Neuroscience*, 106: 131–145.

Higgs, J., Jones, M. A., Loftus, S. and Christensen, N. (2008), *Clinical Reasoning in the Health Professions* (3rd edn.), (Elsevier, Oxford).

Hoffa, A. (1897), *Technik de Massage* (Verlag Von Ferdinand Ernke, Stuttgart).

Holey, E. and Cook, E. (2011), *Evidence-Based Therapeutic Massage* (Elsevier, London).

Hopper, D., Connelly, M. and Chromiak, F. (2005), 'Evaluation of the effect of two massage techniques on hamstring muscle length in competitive female hockey players', *Physical Therapy in Sport*, 6(3): 137–145.

Jones, M. (1992), 'Clinical reasoning in manual therapy', *Physical Therapy*, 72(12): 875–884.

Khan, K. M. and Scott, A. (2009), 'Mechanotherapy: How physical therapists' prescription of exercise promotes tissue repair', *British Journal of Sports Medicine*, 43(4): 247–251.

Lamas, K., Lindholm, L., Stenlund, H., Engstrom, B. and Jacobsson, C. (2009), 'Effects of abdominal massage in management of constipation – a randomized controlled trial', *International Journal of Nursing Studies*, 46(6): 759–767.

LeMoon, K. (2008), 'Clinical reasoning in massage therapy', *International Journal of Therapeutic Massage and Bodywork*, 1(1): 12–18.

Longworth, J. (1982), 'Psychophysiological effects of slow stroke back massage in normotensive females', *Advances in Nursing Science*, 4: 44–61.

Maher, C. G., Latimer, J. and Starkey, I. (2002), 'An evaluation of Superthumb and the Kneeshaw device as manual therapy tools', *Australian Journal of Physiotherapy*, 48(1): 25–30.

Melzack, R. (1975), 'The McGill Pain Questionnaire: Major properties and scoring methods', *Pain*, 1: 277–299.

Mennell, J. B. (1920), *Physical Treatment by Movement, Manipulation and Massage* (Blakiston, Philadelphia).

Morelli, M., Seabourne, D. and Sullivan, S. (1990), 'Changes in H-reflex amplitude during massage of triceps surae in healthy subjects', *Journal of Orthopedics and Sports Physical Therapy*, 12(2): 55–59.

Norris, C. M. (2011), *Managing Sports Injuries* (Elsevier, Oxford).

Paterson, C. (1996), 'Measuring outcomes in primary care: A patient generated measure, MYMOP, compared with the SF-36 health survey', *British Medical Journal*, 312: 1016–1020.

Sacket, D. L., Rosenberg, W. M. C., Gray, J. A. M. and Richardson, W. S. (1996), 'Evidence based medicine: What it is and what it isn't', *British Medical Journal*, 312(1): 71–72.

Seers, K., Crichton, N., Martin, J., Coulson, K. and Carroll, D. (2008), 'A randomised controlled trial to assess the effectiveness of a single session of nurse administered massage for short term relief of chronic non-malignant pain', *BMC Nursing*, July 4: 7–10.

Svedlund, J. et al. (1988), 'GSRS – a clinical rating scale for gastrointestinal symptoms in patients with irritable bowel syndrome and peptic ulcer disease', *Digestive Diseases and Sciences*, 33(2): 129–134.

Taylor, A. G., Galper, D. I., Taylor, P. et al. (2003), 'Effects of adjunctive Swedish massage and vibration therapy on short-term postoperative outcomes: A randomized, controlled trial', *Journal of Alternative and Complementary Medicine*, February 9(1): 77–89.

Weerapong, P. et al. (2005), 'The mechanisms of massage and effects on performance, muscle recovery and injury prevention', *Sports Medicine*, 35(2): 235–256.

# INDEX